# JOG, RUN, RACE

**BOOKS BY JOE HENDERSON**

*Long Slow Distance—The Humane Way to Train (1969)*
*Road Racers and Their Training (1970)*
*Thoughts on the Run (1970)*
*Run Gently Run Long (1974)*
*First Steps to Fitness (1974)*
*Running with Style (1975)*
*Step Up to Racing (1975)*
*The Long Run Solution (1976)*
*Jog, Run, Race (1977)*

# JOG, RUN, RACE

by Joe Henderson

Published by
World Publications

Photography by David Madison


World Publications
P.O. Box 366, Mountain View, CA 94042



Library of Congress: 77-73651
ISBN: 0-89037-121-0 (Hb.), 0-89037-122-9 (Ppb.)

*Second Printing, July 1977*
*Third Printing, November 1977*
*Fourth Printing, April 1978*
*Fifth Printing, August 1978*
*Sixth Printing, October 1978*

*Dedicated to my father, Jim Henderson, and to my brother, Mike, who gave me an early appetite for running which never has waned.*

# Contents

# Schedules and Charts

# Author's Note

A book in progress is almost human. As it grows, it takes a shape and personality of its own, and displays its own emotions apart from the author's.

This is the 11th book or booklet I've written (including two as yet unpublished). And each has been different in the way it grew. Each took shape in ways different from how I'd first visualized them, as if it had a plan I hadn't known. Each found its own style.

This book took a nickname from the way it grew. I called it the "90-Day Wonder"—not because the content was wonderous but because it came together so quickly. (My earlier writings had taken 2-4 times that long to complete.)

It apparently was material meant to come out quickly, because it evolved from thoughts to finished manuscript in three months. There now is something where before there had been only latent ideas eager to be given life on paper.

Like most runners who've been at running a long time and enjoying it, I want others to see the same light and to share this activity from which so many blessings seem to flow. In other words, we're missionaries for running. I try to control my missionary zeal most of the time. But a book like this brings it into full view.

No one talks or writes so enthusiastically as when he is telling someone else what is bad for him. But convincing him of the errors of his ways is only half the job. The other half is outlining a corrective program.

I jump into this eagerly because I'm a frustrated coach. In high school, I tried to convert my teammates to my way of running. No one listened. When I got to college, I trained myself to be a coach. No one wanted to hire me.

I suppose I've coached indirectly through my other writing. But I've never had the chance to outline day-to-day programs. Now I do. I have an audience which needs coaching the most and gets the least, and I've let out everything which has been saved up all this time.

As surely as there is a latent missionary-coach in me, I know there is a runner hidden in almost everyone. He's waiting for the right combination of inspiration and instruction to set him free. Once he's let loose, he can take you places you never imagined going.

In the time it took me to write this book, you can become your own "90-Day Wonder." You can make something where there apparently was nothing before. Ninety days from now, you can have a new set of abilities and habits.

I don't mean to suggest that it will be easy. Creating never is. There may be some very bad days. But promise yourself that you'll last out the full three months and reflect on how far you've come before deciding where to go from there.

Run by steps and measure your progress by miles. Follow the schedules in the book day by day, as I have followed this book's outline point by point in the writing.

Move forward and upward in small steps. Run the prescribed distance or time, as I wrote my assigned number of words each day. A few minutes a day of running or a few hundred words of writing doesn't sound like much. Anyone could handle them. But multiply those small amounts by 90 and you have created something which was there all along but needed some help uncovering itself—something which should keep going and growing past the limits of my preaching and teaching.

If you're starting running for the first time, don't let it bother you that you've never done this kind of thing before. Neither have I, and I'm not bothered. I welcome the chance to make this fresh start.

---

I've never been a beginner in the sense that you probably are. I see the audience for this book as being made up mostly of people my age. The last time you were in good shape was during high school, and your 10th class reunion has come and gone. Your college studies, new career and growing family have taken precedence over physical activity during those years.

You're now looking, to put it in a charitable word, "prosperous." You're hiding the growing bulge around your belt line behind expensive camouflage.

As the bulge has grown, so has the nagging voice in the back of your mind. It says, "You really should be getting some exercise."

You have answered, "I would. But I just don't have time for it. Maybe later."

Now, finally, you're making the time.

I've never had a paunch because I've always made the time to run. I say I've never been a true beginner because I started formal running at the age of 14, when I was still a child who unconsciously had been training to be a runner since my first steps. I haven't stopped running for more than a month at a time in the last 20 years.

I don't say this to imply, "Look how much better I am than you." I say it to point out only that we are different. In a way, you're stronger than I am because you're willing to suffer the pains of reconditioning yourself to exercise. This takes much more effort than my continuing to do what I've always done. The initially painful and ultimately rewarding experience you're having now is one I've never known.

My background is in competitive running. I raced, hard, through high school and college. And I still race on a low level from time to time. Competition has values and beauties of its own, and I recommend that you sample them sometime. But if you're in your 20s or 30s or beyond, don't start with it as a main goal. It will get you into trouble by leading to extremes.

I ran to extremes for my first 10 years, going too fast and too far. I hurt myself physically and, worse, I lost my appetite for more running.

Running couldn't do me any good if I wasn't able or willing

to keep it up. (Its benefits don't last long and must be renewed several times a week.) So I systematically "unlearned" most of the lessons of training for competition. I intentionally ran at a gentle pace. I seldom, if ever, pushed myself hard enough to hurt. I ran distances which were quite small when looked at for a single day, but which added up to a lot over the weeks, months and years that I kept going.

The secret to good running is simply to keep going. And the way to keep at it is to keep the distances and paces modest, and to keep healthy and happy.

While I may not have shared your experience of being a beginner, I have learned something about this basic principle of running which applies to all of us. This, I think, gives a solid foundation to my preaching and teaching.

You and I probably are similar in another way besides not having been beginners. I doubt that you've ever read a book like this before. That's okay, because I've never written one.

My other 10 books were for myself and people like me. They were written for the old-timers of running who didn't really need books–not instructional books, anyway. They already were running, and would have kept right on running without reading about it.

The other 10 books were "thought" books, intended to solidify the thinking and strengthen the biases of runners who'd had some of the same thoughts themselves. I wrote in generalities, intending for readers to sketch in their own specifics. I was offering the "whys," and it was up to them to supply their own "hows." This assumed that the readers had the experience to draw their own conclusions on just how they should put my vague ideas into practice.

Here, I assume that you never have run before and that you know nothing about the guiding principles of running. This may or may not be true. But chances are if you've had experiences, they have been the wrong ones. Otherwise, you wouldn't be turning to this book for advice. Forget what you might have done in running before, or heard or read about it, and make a fresh start.

---

Commit yourself to the three months of running I recommend here. After that much time, you'll know whether you're meant to be a runner or not. You will have experienced enough of its joys and despairs, pleasures and pains to decide whether or not to continue.

Why three months? Runners on all levels know that it takes about two months of training to build a solid conditioning base from which to move to a higher plane of fitness. I allow an extra month as a break-in period.

When to start? The year-round runner in me says, "No time is better than right now." Realistically, though, I know you won't be eager to step outside for the first time in sub-zero cold and snow, or in 100-degree humid heat.

The solution may be to start with the coming of spring, the traditional time for new beginnings—or to begin with autumn, when the best running weather of the year arrives. Run through the season, and your new momentum may carry you into the next, less pleasant one.

What to run? This is the purpose of the book—to tell you what to do and how to do it. Basically, what I'm asking you to invest from the start is about a half-hour of your time at least every other day. (I use the word "invest" because your eventual return should far exceed the time and effort spent.)

I ask one more thing which I've never asked of my readers before. Follow the training schedules I've outlined. I haven't forced them upon experienced runners because they are capable of making their own plans. You will be too—later.

But now you're groping with new information and routines. The schedules are maps to follow until you know the territory. They aren't sacred, so don't hesitate to modify the suggested routes. But you'll save yourself a lot of miles if you go more or less in the recommended direction.

# PART ONE

# STARTING

# Lesson 1

# Run, Don't Read

"Whenever I feel the urge to exercise, I lie down until it goes away."

I don't know who first said that. And when I had the urge to look up the exact words and who uttered them, I laid down until it passed. But whoever it was, he has lots of people practicing his advice.

This is why I start by saying don't sit there any longer thinking, "It's time I started doing something to get in shape." Because the longer you think about it, the more time you give the urge to pass.

Don't think about it any longer. Do it.

Don't check with your doctor to see if it's okay. By the time he says it is, it may be too late.

Don't take time to plan what you'll do. Just plan to start, now, and let what happens happen.

Don't pay any attention to the advisors on exercise who say, "Be cautious." Jump into it with both feet.

Don't go out first and buy new shoes and clothes. The urge to exercise may die before you get back home, and the $25 striped green shoes and $40 stretch nylon warmups will remain to haunt you.

Don't wait. Run while you feel like it, in the way you think you should. Do it on the track or on the street. Sprint or jog or combine the two. Race the clock, or race an imaginary opponent, or try to finish a distance you've set for yourself. Do whatever you want, but do it.

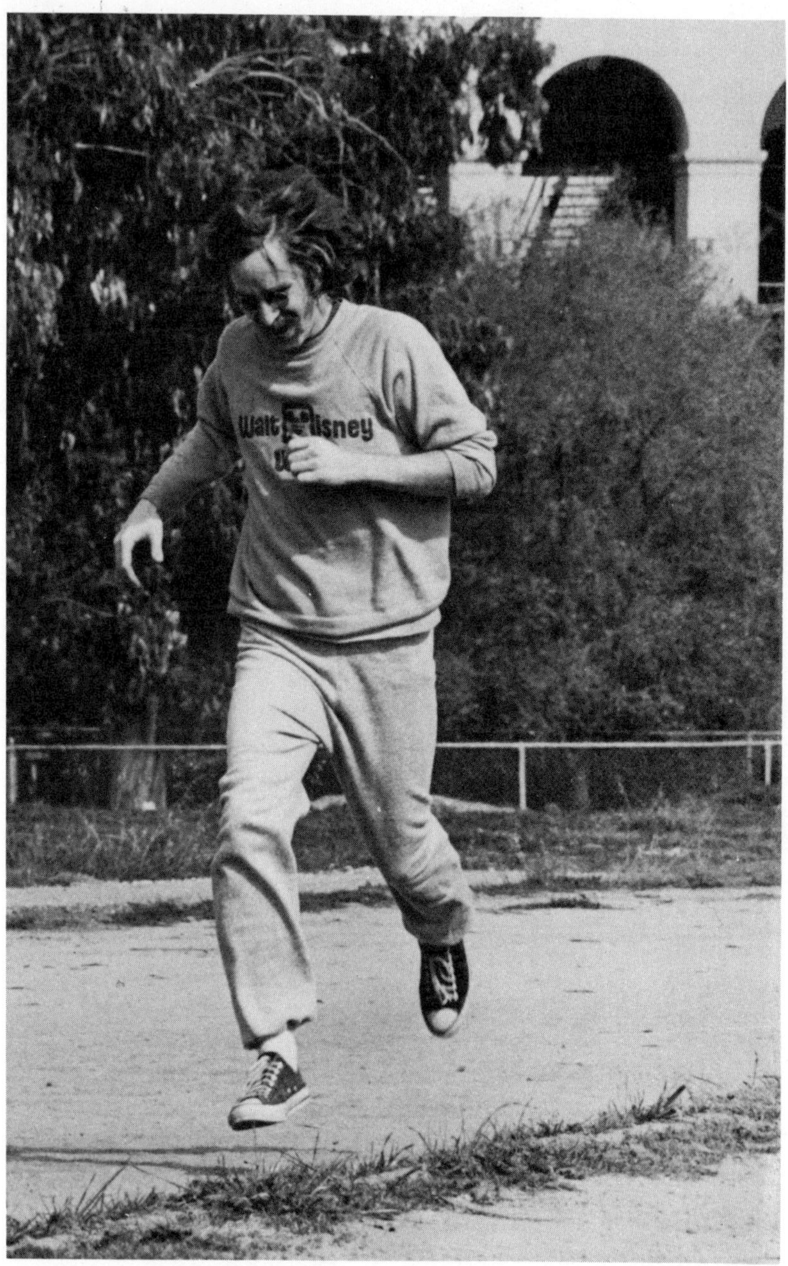

*"Most new runners start like this—in a sudden explosion of enthusiasm and not by a rational, conservative, guided plan. Some of them get hurt . . . ."*

This may not be the ideal way to start running. Each of the last six paragraphs contains advice which experts on exercise will tell you is dead wrong. I'm not saying it is completely right, either. I'm only saying this is the way it is, and maybe the way it should be.

Most new runners start like this—in a sudden explosion of enthusiasm and not by a rational, conservative, guided plan. Sure, they make mistakes. Some of them get hurt. But it should be a basic right of man to be free to make his own mistakes, to hurt himself in any way he sees fit.

The first run is almost guaranteed to be painful, and right now I'm neither telling you how to avoid that pain or that you should try to avoid it.

Pain can be a good teacher. It can force lessons on you which you never would have noticed had the run been easy and pleasant. Later, you'll make adjustments based on these lessons, and you'll know exactly why you're making them, since avoidance of pain is one of man's basic drives.

All I ask here in this first lesson is that you don't try to be a hero. Once your legs start to ache and your breath starts to come in burning waves, don't be too proud to stop. Your body is trying to tell you something. Its early-warning system is working, and you can't do yourself any serious damage if you listen to it.

# Lesson 2

# Look Back

I wanted you to start your own way, to make your own mistakes, in order to get your attention. You'll now remember what was wrong about that first run, and will use it as grounds for setting things right.

You won't soon forget that first time. The worse it was—the more embarrassed you felt, the harder your illusions about your physical abilities fell, the worse you labored—the better you'll remember the first run.

You probably won't remember it with pleasure. It's likely you hated nearly every step of it, and you flinch when you think and talk about it. But you keep thinking and talking because you can't get it out of your mind. Later, you'll bore people with the gory details which don't fade with time but are embellished as the memories age.

My first serious run was nearly 20 years ago. It was a mile race, and I remember it as if it happened last week. Its details are imprinted on my brain as vividly as the picture of what I was doing when the news came that Kennedy had been shot. I remember more about that race than about my most recent one.

I remember the place (Tarkio, Mo.), the name of the meet (Tri-State Relays), the date (April 2, 1958), the weather (gray, cold and windy), the way I felt (confident that I would place among the top five), the condition of the track (cinders the size of golf balls, tufts of dead grass on the backstretch).

I remember where I lined up at the start of that race (second

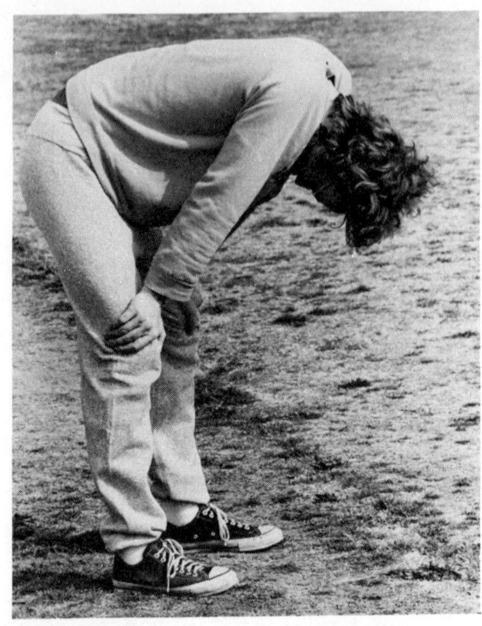

*"You won't soon forget that first time. The worse it was, the better you'll remember the first run . . . ."*

lane, second row), how I started (banged from elbow to elbow like a loose hockey puck), where I was when the shoving stopped (third from last), the first quarter-mile time (70 seconds), where I dropped out (on the first turn of the second lap, where no one was standing), how I reacted (I never wanted to take another running step).

There obviously have been uncounted millions of running steps since then, and nearly 600 more races. None of them has left anything like the same lasting impressions as that first aborted mile.

I could have quit running then, almost before I'd started. I came very close to quitting, but my coach and my brother said the right things at the right time.

The coach said, "There's nothing wrong with you that a little training won't cure." I hadn't known that runners did anything besides race.

My brother said, "There's nothing wrong with you that a little pace judgment won't correct." I had thought that running was simply going as fast as you could for as far as you could.

I'd run without preparing and without pacing myself that first time. It had been a disaster, and one I wouldn't forget. But I'm happy now that my running started that way.

That race told me what I'd done wrong, what I didn't want to repeat and how to start over again with a more cautious and realistic plan. I never could have learned so much from a successful start.

This is why I told you in Lesson One to run however you felt like running—to make your own mistakes. There's no better way to imprint on your mind how you *shouldn't* run than to experience it. That early lesson will make the ones to come easier to understand and accept. You'll know now the reasons for them.

Let's review Lesson One. This is what you probably did wrong:

1. No pre-run checkout and clearance, either formally from a doctor or by realistically evaluating your own condition and limits. (Lesson Four tells you how to make up your own "Personal Fitness Scorecard," and to find a starting level based on your score.)

2. No advice from anyone on what you should or shouldn't try to do; or if you had advice, you ignored it. (This book is full of such advice. Pay particular attention to the odd-numbered lessons from 11 on.)

3. No plan on how far or how fast you were to go; you simply thought, "I'll run till I don't feel like running any more," and that end came much sooner than you expected. (Throughout the book are specific day-by-day schedules telling just how much to attempt.)

In short, you took your first run on impulse, just as I suggested you should have (and you would have without my suggestion). You ran to extremes and likely suffered a bit for it.

Fine. Now back off. Start over again the right way, by learning the reasons why the first run didn't go so well and by practicing some restraint.

Restraint, holding back a little bit, stopping short. These are key concepts in running. Distance running is a process of rationing out effort, of intentionally running at something less than your best effort so you are able to keep going for a longer time.

Three things a new runner must learn before going any farther are (1) the ability to *plan* efforts which spread available energy over the distance to be covered; (2) a feeling for the right *pace* while going that distance, and (3) the *patience* to last out the distance.

Consider the following suggestions as you plan your running:

- Find your own current level of fitness (see Lesson Four).
- Match your present limits with the appropriate type of training (walking, jogging, running, racing).
- Decide how far you want to progress (walking to jogging, jogging to running, etc.).
- Move one step at a time toward that goal (following the schedules in the lessons starting with six).

Later, there will be more spontaneity and speed in your running program. But in the beginning, I ask you to go by the book and to hold yourself back. Follow a plan until you can trust your instincts to keep you on a sensible course. Be able to walk long distances before running them, and run the distances slowly before thinking of racing them.

# Lesson 3

# Start Over

A basic law of physics is that a body's natural tendency is to stay at rest when it's resting and to stay in motion when it's moving. This applies to the human body, same as all others.

One of the greatest accomplishments and curses of 20th century technology is that it has eliminated most self-propelled movement, making it voluntary instead of required.

The strange twist in this shift is that as we are required to do less moving on foot, we need it more than ever. Our legs and hearts and heads are made to move, and decay sets in when they don't get the movement they need.

But this is where the inertia problem comes in. A person doesn't readily do what he isn't forced to do. When he can rest behind the wheel of a car or in front of the TV, he tends to stay at rest there. The less he moves—the less exercise he gives his legs, heart and head—the less he is able to move. The effort of moving grows in inverse relationship to the amount of it he does—until finally he must make a great effort to move the few feet from the easy chair to the garage and the parking lot to the office.

Talking of jogging-running in abstract terms, viewing it from a distance, it appears to offer all sorts of attractive results. It appeals to the egotist in all of us who wants to look and feel young forever. It promises glowing health, abundant energy and a relaxed personality.

But to have any of these, you must take the first step. You must break the powerful hold of resting inertia which has you rooted to one spot. You must start moving, and that starting may be one of the hardest things you ever do.

I once wrote, "Running is easy, but starting running is not. The first steps are never easy." I was speaking for myself and echoing what other runners have said.

Ron Clarke, an Australian who set dozens of world records in the 1960s, said then that the only hard thing about running was putting on his shoes and forcing himself out the door.

George Young, the first American to run in four Olympic Games, said, "There is nothing hard about running the hundred miles a week that I do. Almost anyone could do it. The hard part is making yourself roll out of bed in the morning and start running."

These athletes get up and out because they've done it so long they don't know how else to start a day. They know that once they're in motion, they'll stay in motion.

A beginner doesn't know these things. His habits are in the direction of resting inertia, not moving, so his start is immensely more difficult to make than that of a runner who practices overcoming the laws of physics daily.

Assuming you've caught the vision of what running has to offer, the task now is to turn that vision into forward motion.

Don't dream any more. Do! And once you start doing, don't think too much because you might start thinking up more reasons for *not* running than for continuing.

Be warned that the vision dims quickly when it bangs up against the day-to-day realities of putting your feet in your running shoes and moving yourself out the door.

The first day may be relatively easy. You're still fresh, eager and full of the vision. But then the second day is harder than the first, the third is harder yet. You see no progress toward the promised land. In fact, you're farther from it than when you were doing nothing at all.

Running was supposed to trim off weight faster than a day in the steam bath, but the scales say you've *gained* two pounds.

The new activity was said to tap energy sources you never knew you had, but you're falling in bed at 9:30 for nine hours of dreamless sleep.

You were promised new strength and tone in your leg muscles, but you're shuffling along with the gait of an 80-year-old arthritic on legs which are one big pain from the knees down.

You thought you were the athlete of your youth. You ignored the warning, "Start very slowly. Walk if you must." You timed yourself for a mile on the track the first day, and it took nine minutes and 55 seconds. You tried again the second day, and the time was more than 10 minutes. You won't talk about your time the third day.

Yesterday, you were too sore to face a run first thing in the morning. You told yourself, "I'll sneak it in before dinner. I'll feel better by then." Then you found reasons to be delayed at the office. It was nearly dark when you got home, and dinner was ready. "Can't keep the family waiting for me," you said.

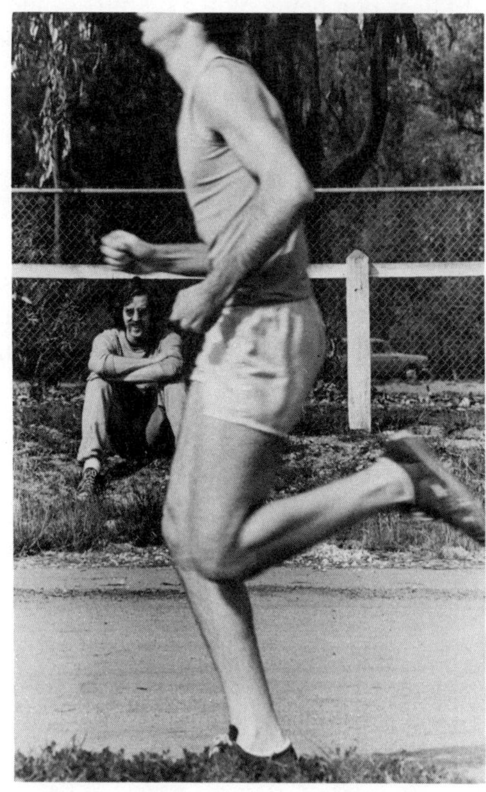

*"Running promises glowing health, abundant energy and a relaxed personality. But to have these, you must take the first step . . . ."*

"Besides, it isn't safe to run at night with all the cars and muggers on the streets."

This morning, the alarm jolts you awake at 6:30. You think, "Good, I can sleep another half-hour or so." But as you roll back over and pull the covers over your head, you remember: "Run!" And you groan. You must leave the warm peace of the bed for a romp in the icy outdoors.

You rifle through your sleepy head for reasons why you shouldn't go out. You want excuses to avoid this awful shock to your system.

You test your legs by flexing the knees and ankles in bed, hoping to find a compound fracture.

You swallow, hoping the first stages of the flu might have settled in your throat during the night.

You listen for sounds outside the bedroom window, hoping to hear rain being blown by hurricane-force winds.

You peek over the edge of the bed, hoping the dog has gnawed the uppers off your new nylon Adidas.

Anything to keep from moving.

You're facing a crisis. Every runner faces it every day to a certain extent as he goes from resting to moving. But for the veteran, the effort of breaking resting inertia is equal to pedaling a bicycle away from a stop sign. For a beginner, it seems more like pushing a stalled Mack truck up a slight incline by hand. It's hard as hell to contemplate, but something to be proud of once it's accomplished. At this stage, simply starting is a major victory.

# Lesson 4

# Test Yourself

Every book on exercise, every program outlined in a magazine, begins with a warning: "First, get your doctor's okay."

This makes you wonder right away, "What kind of danger am I putting myself into if I require a medical dispensation?"

Maybe the writers of these books and articles feel they would be held liable in case of accidents. So they shift the blame to the doctors, or to the individual who ignores the first order. Whatever the reason, the warning is always included–and nearly always ignored.

I don't include it for several reasons–the least of which is that most of you would pay no attention even if I told you to see your doctor first. I don't want you starting with the idea that you're likely to do yourself damage or even die from running. And this is the message the medical warning which implies: "Caution: Exercise may be hazardous to your health."

Doctors are trained, and in most cases trained quite well, in the diagnosis and treatment of injury and disease. They can tell you quickly and clearly how hurt or ill you are, and what to do to get better. They are well equipped to help you back to health, but they are less sure of themselves when it comes to achieving fitness.

Fitness is a step above health. Health is the mere absence of disease and injury, while fitness is the ability to perform physically. You can be healthy and not fit, but you can't be fit without first being healthy.

A doctor can certify by scanning your records, listening to

your heart and measuring your blood pressure that you are alive and well. He can tell you that you have the *basis* for developing fitness, but unless he is a runner or similar athlete himself he can't be considered an expert on exercise.

(This is the typical family doctor I'm talking about. There are a growing number of facilities around the country, notably Dr. Kenneth Cooper's Aerobics Center in Dallas, which evaluate both health and fitness. They do elaborate testing and prescribe supervised exercise programs based on the test results. However, most beginners won't have access to this type of service—and indeed don't need anything this advanced.)

If you visit your doctor, one of two things is likely to happen:

1. He'll tell you what you already know—that "nothing is wrong with you and I see no reason why you shouldn't exercise," or that "your blood pressure (or cholesterol, or weight) is a little high, and you should be careful about overdoing it."

2. He'll tell you what you don't want to hear. He'll say, "Why would someone your age want to do something like that? There's no medical reason not to do it, but there's also no proof that it does any good."

Not all doctors are sold on the idea of vigorous exercise. Many are cautious about prescribing it. A few are outwardly hostile to the idea and will say, "I can never give my approval to anything so foolish."

This is why I say a medical checkup is optional. It may confirm your good opinion about your health, but you may also end up running against doctor's orders.

The doctor may give you some idea about where to start. But the more important information in that area must come from an evaluation you give yourself.

You should know better than anyone about the workings of this body you've lived in all these years. You should know how it feels, what is right and wrong with it, what it can and can't do. So who should know better than you if it is capable of accepting a running program and, if so, what type?

Be honest with yourself. Because if you aren't honest now,

the running you try to do will uncover your lies later. Look closely at yourself, your habits and capabilities. Decide which ones contribute to and detract from your potential as a runner.

Be honest now. Are you really all the athlete you were 20 years ago when you ran high school cross-country? Has that nine holes of golf once a week really kept you in shape? Is that breathlessness you feel at the top of the stairs really due to the altitude? Have you "filled out" since college, or is that just fat you've put on? Is it true that "a couple of cigarettes a day won't hurt me"? Be honest.

Rate yourself on the accompanying scorecard to determine how fit you are now and how you realistically should begin exercising–at a walk, a jog or a run.

The first four tests are the most important. The first three may stop you from going further in this book even if you can pass all the others. The fourth may let you go ahead even as the tests after it say "hold back."

1. **Do you have any diagnosed heart or circulatory problems?** Coronary disease? Chronic chest pains? Extremely high cholesterol readings? High blood pressure? Prior heart attack or heart surgery?

If you say yes to any of these, find other help. I'm not saying you can't exercise. Exercise is an important tool in controlling and correcting these problems. But you need a well-supervised program such as the cardiac rehabilitation classes offered by many YMCAs.

I frankly don't want the responsibility of guiding you by way of a book if you have any of these problems. The risk is too great. I've already seen one man too many die at my feet.

He was a 46-year-old. One warm Sunday morning, he ran 7½ miles at top speed. He collapsed of a heart attack 50 yards from the finish and never woke up. His wife said later that he had a history of high blood pressure.

It is impossible to damage a healthy heart with any amount or severity of exercise. However, unhealthy hearts do give out under stress. If you suspect something is wrong with yours, find better guidance than I can give.

Two more medical questions come next. They aren't as critical as the first one because they aren't life-and-death matters. You don't need to solicit a doctor's advice on them, but you must ask them of yourself.

2. **Are there any injuries which might slow or stop you, or which running might aggravate?**

This question is directed particularly at the feet and legs. Do you have an old ankle sprain which still gives you trouble? Do your arches ache when you've been on your feet a long time? Are you inclined to develop shin splints when you exercise vigorously? Does your knee still give you trouble from a high school football injury?

You'll have to adjust your activity to your aches and pains, both now and for as long as you run, because running works in strange ways. It corrects many chronic problems by strengthening the legs. However, it also produces some new pains of its own.

All runners get sore. But the old-timers of the sport say, "An injury is serious only if it keeps me from running."

Rate the seriousness of an injury according to how much it limits activity.

3. **Do you have any illnesses (other than those listed in question one) which might limit you?**

This includes both acute conditions such as colds and the flu, and chronic ones like allergies, asthma and diabetes.

Adjust for them the same way you do for injuries. And judge them by the same standard: How much or how little will they allow you to do?

This is probably the most important question of all:

4. **How did your first run go?**

This is assuming you took Lesson One and are still here to talk about it. (If you're running now, base this question on your most recent run.) The real test is how well you can run. All those which follow are contributors to fitness, signs of it or detractors from it. If you can run well, nothing else can be too badly wrong.

If you went a half-mile or more (five mi were going by time instead of distance) th much strain and without having to walk, y directly into the jogging schedule (Lesson N the other indicators say.

If you made 1½ miles or 15 minutes ready for more advanced running (Lesson 1 , ,.

However, if you had to stop short of a half-mile or five minutes, you probably need a refresher course in how to move on foot, starting with some walking.

The rest of the tests, looked at separately or as a group, are good measures of your potential to run and are good indicators of how you should approach running. The next two relate to the experience you've had before which might prepare you to run now.

5. **Have you ever been a runner?**

Of course everyone has been a runner, and still is a latent one, because running is a basic form of human movement. We all ran as children, but most people have run since then only when they absolutely had to.

What I really have in mind in this question is, "Have you had any *formal* running training since you were a teenager?" Have you followed a regular program which allowed you to go long distances rather comfortably, or to run shorter distances at high speeds?

The condition you were in then disappeared quickly once you stopped training. But the memory of how that running felt and how it was accomplished was much slower to fade. If you still have the memory of running well, you probably have an advantage over those who never have run. The closer you are to your past as a runner, the more advantage you have.

6. **What other sports or physical activities do you practice now?**

You may just be a short step away from running without realizing it. Do you commute to work and back on a bike? Do you walk a lot on weekdays and take back-packing trips on and vacations? Do you swim laps in the pool just for of it?

so, you've laid the groundwork for running. While fitness m one activity doesn't transfer perfectly to another, all of these are closely related to running. Biking, hiking and swimming all are steady, drawn-out, so-called "endurance" or "aerobic" sports. And you're already in excellent shape if you practice them regularly. Perhaps more importantly, you're preconditioned to *thinking* like an endurance athlete.

The stop-and-go sports aren't so valuable in this way, but still indicate a certain disposition toward running. These include tennis, basketball, soccer and possibly football—though I tend to lump football with the next group of sports.

The slow sports: football, baseball, softball and golf. In these, more time is spent standing than moving, and as such they contribute only marginally to endurance fitness. Still, they're better than the nothing many adults do.

Three more questions deal with numbers which each give a good general idea of your physical standing:

7. **How old are you?** Age takes a physical toll not because the years alone are adding up, but because of the years of *neglect and inactivity* during that time. The years from the mid-20s to the mid-30s have been labeled the "dangerous decade" because this is when youthful activity usually slips away and the sedentary habits of the rest of one's life set in. Physical fitness declines faster during this period than at any other comparable time.

It's never too late to reclaim some of your youthful vigor. But the farther you are from youth when you start, and the longer you've been inactive, the longer and harder this climb back to fitness will be.

8. **How much do you weigh?**

If you're rather lightly built, imagine putting on a 25-pound backpack and running a mile with it. Think how much harder the run would be.

If you're heavy, imagine the opposite—that your extra weight suddenly can be taken off like a pack. Don't you feel a lot better as you run now?

Since you must lift your full weight off the ground with each running step, it's reasonable to assume that the lighter you are the easier you'll run. People who already are at or near their ideal weight have a big headstart in the sport.

What is ideal? You can check the weight charts published almost everywhere, but they aren't much good because they deal with averages—and the average person is overweight.

You can use Dr. Irwin Stillman's formula: (men) 110 pounds plus 5½ pounds for each inch over five feet; (women) 100 pounds plus five pounds for each inch over five feet. But he, too, is dealing with people who are typical in structure.

Another rule of thumb is that your ideal weight probably was what you weighed on your 20th birthday—after you'd finished growing up and before you started growing out. Anything you've put on since then probably is fat. But this doesn't account for people who've always carried too much weight.

Somehow, determine your "ideal" and remember that fatness and fitness don't go together.

9. **What is your resting pulse rate?**

A strong heart beats slowly because it is efficient. It does more work per beat than a weaker heart. Therefore, a slow pulse rate is a healthy sign.

"Normal" pulse is 70-75. But this norm, like the one for weight, is an average—and the average heart is untrained. Moderately trained runners usually have pulse rates in the 50s, and the better athletes' hearts plod along at rates in the 40s or lower.

The final question has to do with the single habit which does the most immediate and profound damage to the type of health and fitness running tries to promote.

10. **Do you smoke?** If you smoke heavily, cut down. If you smoke occasionally, try to stop. If you've stopped, work on correcting the lingering effects. If you've never smoked, count yourself as one of the lucky ones.

## Fitness Scorecard

**1. CARDIOVASCULAR HEALTH*** __________

0—under medical care for heart or circulatory problems.

1—such problems exist but medical care not required.

2—past cardiovascular ailments have been pronounced "cured."

3—no history of cardiovascular trouble.

**2. INJURIES**** __________

0—unable to do any strenuous work because of an injury.

1—level of activity is limited by the injury.

2—some pain during activity but performance isn't affected significantly.

3—no injuries.

**3. ILLNESSES**** __________

0—unable to do any strenuous work because of an illness.

1—level of activity is limited by the illness.

2—some during activity but performance isn't affected significantly.

3—no illnesses.

**4. FIRST (OR MOST RECENT) RUN***** __________

0—able to run less than a half-mile or five minutes without stopping.

1—ran between a half-mile and a mile (5-10 minutes) non-stop the first time.

2—completed between a mile and 1½ miles (10-15 minutes) the first time.

3—went more than 1½ miles or 15 continuous minutes.

**5. RUNNING BACKGROUND** __________

0—have never trained formally for running.

1—no running training within the last three years or more.

2—no running training within the last 1-2 years.

3—have trained for running within the last year.

**6. OTHER RELATED ACTIVITIES** __________

0—not currently active in any regular sports or exercise programs.

1—regularly participate in "slow sports" such as golf, baseball, softball, football.

2—regularly practice vigorous "stop-and-go" sports such as tennis, basketball, soccer.

3—regularly participate in steady-paced, prolonged activities such as bicycling, hiking, swimming.

**7. AGE** __________

0—50s and older

1—40s.

2—30s.

3—20s or younger

**8. WEIGHT** __________

0—more than 25 pounds above your "ideal" weight.

1—16-25 pounds above your "ideal" weight.

2—6-15 pounds above your "ideal" weight.

3—within five pounds of "ideal" weight (or below ideal weight).

**9. RESTING PULSE RATE** __________

0—80 beats per minute or higher.

1—in the 70s.

2—in the 60s.

3—in the 50s or below.

**10. SMOKING** __________

0—a regular smoker.

1—an occasional smoker.

2—have been a regular smoker but quit.

3—never have smoked regularly.

Score yourself in each of the 10 areas and add up the total:

**TOTAL SCORE:** _____

A score of 20 or higher is excellent. You probably can skip the preliminaries and go directly to a *running* program (Lesson 17).

A score of 10-19 is average for adults. Start at the *jogging* level (Lesson Nine).

If you scored less than 10 points, you should forget about running and even jogging for now and concentrate on raising your score by *walking* (Lesson Five).

Exceptions:

* = If you have any history of heart or circulatory disease, do not continue with this book's programs; participate only in closely supervised activities.

** = If these injuries or illnesses are temporary, wait until they are cured before starting the programs; if they're chronic, adjust the programs to fit your limitations.

*** = If you can run continuously for 1½ miles (15 minutes) or more, you may start as high as the running program (Lesson 17) no matter what your score is; you are fit!

# PART TWO

# WALKING

# Lesson 5

# Introducing Walking

Walk. Just walk. Don't even think about jogging or running for now if you can count your fitness score from Lesson Four on two hands. If your score was less than 10, your first objective is simply to get back on your feet.

It isn't an admission of defeat to start by walking. Instead, it's an honest recognition of the fact that you aren't very fit and that you must start slowly. In a way, this is a bigger victory than that of someone who is moving from jogging to running or running to racing. He's just increasing the amount and intensity of what he already was doing. But you're shifting from doing nothing to doing something.

You're doing it in the wisest way possible, by working into it gradually. Just as you wouldn't race the engine of a car which has sat idle in the driveway all winter without first tuning and warming it up, you don't ask a body which hasn't worked hard in years to race before it is prepared.

The idea now is to break yourself in to exercise without breaking yourself down. Strengthen your legs without pounding them too hard. Make your heart work without making it pound too hard. Lay the groundwork for a new habit of everyday exercise without making yourself sick and tired of it.

You can accomplish all of this by walking. This is the type of walking I propose for the first month:

Make no big deal of it. Follow no formal plan, do no special preparations for it and buy no special equipment. Just start walking.

Set aside a half-hour at least every other day for your walk. You might go a mile or two, but for God's sake don't time yourself. Walk for a certain period of time or a certain distance, but don't combine time and distance or you'll end up racing yourself. That isn't the idea now. You want to walk along resolutely, with purpose, but at a non-exhausting pace.

Combine your walk with activities which already need doing. Get up a little earlier in the morning and go for a walk with the dog. Or park the car a mile or so away from the office, and walk there and back. Or at noon, walk to and from a restaurant a similar distance away, and eat less than usual while you're there. Or walk to the grocery store instead of driving there.

Set some modest goals for the month, and keep a record in the accompanying chart to see how well you achieve them:

- Walk at least 14 days this month—the more the better.

- Walk steadily for at least 20-30 minutes on each of those days.

- If you're overweight, aim at losing five pounds during the month. Weigh yourself daily and watch the amount you eat.

- Make it your goal to feel more relaxed and energetic after a walk than when you started.

## First Month's Walking Plan

| Day | Suggested Training | Actual Training |
|---|---|---|
| 1 | 30-minute walk* | |
| 2 | extra exercise** | |
| 3 | 30-minute walk | |
| 4 | extra exercise | |
| 5 | 30-minute walk | |
| 6 | extra exercise | |
| 7 | 30-minute walk | |
| *Weight at end of first week:* | | |
| 8 | extra exercise | |
| 9 | 30-minute walk | |
| 10 | extra exercise | |
| 11 | 30-minute walk | |
| 12 | extra exercise | |
| 13 | 30-minute walk | |
| 14 | extra exercise | |
| *Weight at end of second week:* | | |

| Day | Suggested Training | Actual Training |
|---|---|---|
| 15 | 30-minute walk | |
| 16 | extra exercise | |
| 17 | 30-minute walk | |
| 18 | extra exercise | |
| 19 | 30-minute walk | |
| 20 | extra exercise | |
| 21 | 30-minute walk | |
| *Weight at end of third week:* | | |
| 22 | extra exercise | |
| 23 | 30-minute walk | |
| 24 | extra exercise | |
| 25 | 30-minute walk | |
| 26 | extra exercise | |
| 27 | 30-minute walk | |
| 28 | extra exercise | |
| *Weight at end of fourth week:* | | |

| Day | Suggested Training | Actual Training |
|---|---|---|
| 29 | makeup day*** | |
| 30 | makeup day | |
| 31 | makeup day | |

*Total number of walking days this month (14):* ______________

*Net weight loss or gain for the month:* ______________________

(*walk at a brisk and steady pace, and don't attempt any jogging or running; **"extra exercise" means increasing the amount of normal daily activity—riding a bike to the store instead of driving, walking up steps instead of taking the elevator, walking to lunch instead of taking the car, etc.; ***walk a "makeup" half-hour on one or two of these days if the total of the month's walking sessions is less than 14)

# Lesson 6

# Build Up

It's a new month and time to move to a new and higher level of exercise. This is a first look at a pattern which repeats itself throughout the book. Whether you're walking, jogging, running or racing, the general plan is the same:

- A three-month program, preferably covering one season of the year (spring and fall are the most friendly to effort of this type).
- First month—a gentle break-in to new and unaccustomed activity.
- Second month—a steady build-up in the amount of activity.
- Third month—leveling off or decreasing the amount and increasing the speed or intensity of training.

I'll assume you've gone through the first break-in month of walking, or that you found it to be much too easy and you've skipped ahead. (If by chance it seemed harder than you expected, repeat it. The idea is for you to be in this program for life once you start, so there's no advantage to rushing ahead.)

Last month, you walked pretty much as the spirit moved you. This month, you graduate to a more formal schedule. It is meant to insure that you progress steadily, and that you have a goal each day to help you make that progress.

Starting now, you are training like a runner. You still are walking and don't want to try running yet. But the day-to-day schedule you're asked to follow is just like that of a runner.

It now involves doing something every day of the week, if

only a short stroll on the easy days. It includes three big days a week in which you may be out for as long as an hour. It recommends that you now buy a good pair of running shoes (see Lesson Eight for details) and that you wear clothes suited for longer walks.

Walk steadily and briskly—no racing the clock, but not dragging your feet and stopping to smell the roses, either. Work up to the point where you can walk the equivalent of a mile of running. This takes quite a bit longer—both in time and distance—with walking. Dr. Kenneth Cooper estimates in his book *Aerobics* that walking is only about one-fourth as strenuous as running. Therefore, you must walk about four times as far to get the same benefit.

This is why I'm setting a four-mile or one-hour walk (don't combine distance and time; walk either the distance or the time, but don't time yourself over a measured distance) as the main goal of this month.

Other goals:

- Make daily walking a habit by doing it nearly every day. Aim at 20 days or more for the month, and an average of a half-hour walk each day.
- Continue to keep tabs on your weight. Weigh yourself each morning before eating and record it. If you're still overweight, try to lose five more pounds this month.
- Check your resting (before training) pulse occasionally. A drop in the heart rate indicates that your fitness is improving.
- Make each week's distance or time total a little higher than the one before.

# Second Month's Walking Plan

| Day | Suggested Training | Actual Training |
|---|---|---|
| 1 | 30-minute walk* | |
| 2 | extra exercise** | |
| 3 | 15-minute walk | |
| 4 | 30-minute walk | |
| 5 | 15-minute walk | |
| 6 | extra exercise | |
| 7 | 40-minute walk | |
| *Weight at end of first week:*<br>*Resting pulse rate:* | | |
| 8 | extra exercise | |
| 9 | 20-minute walk | |
| 10 | 35-minute walk | |
| 11 | extra exercise | |
| 12 | 35-minute walk | |
| 13 | 20-minute walk | |
| 14 | 45-minute walk | |
| *Weight at end of second week:*<br>*Resting pulse rate:* | | |

| Day | Suggested Training | Actual Training |
|---|---|---|
| 15 | extra exercise | |
| 16 | 20-minute walk | |
| 17 | 40-minute walk | |
| 18 | extra exercise | |
| 19 | 40-minute walk | |
| 20 | 20-minute walk | |
| 21 | 50-minute walk | |
| *Weight at end of third week:*<br>*Resting pulse rate:* | | |
| 22 | extra exercise | |
| 23 | 20-minute walk | |
| 24 | 40-minute walk | |
| 25 | extra exercise | |
| 26 | 40-minute walk | |
| 27 | 20-minute walk | |
| 28 | One-hour walk | |
| *Weight at end of fourth week:*<br>*Resting pulse rate:* | | |

| Day | Suggested Training | Actual Training |
|---|---|---|
| 29 | makeup day*** | |
| 30 | makeup day | |
| 31 | makeup day | |

*Total number of walking days this month (20):* ______________

*Net weight loss or gain for the month:* ______________

*Net rise or fall in resting pulse rate:* ______________

(*walk at a brisk and steady pace, and don't attempt any jogging or running; **"extra exercise" means increasing the amount of normal daily activity—walking, bicycling, swimming, etc.; ***make up for one or two of the sessions missed during the month)

# Lesson 7

# Speed Up

You're now used to being on your feet after two months of pure walking. You've had a "break-in" month and a "build-up" month. If you've followed the schedules up till now, you have walked more days than not. You have walked continuously for an hour at a brisk, steady pace. You have lost some weight and gained some strength in your legs and heart. You have started to form an exercise habit.

Your persistence and patience are about to be rewarded. This month you step up to running. Well, actually it's jogging, barely faster than a walk. And most of the training this month still is walking. But this jogging does represent a step up, because finally you are breaking contact with the ground.

I'm introducing you here to "intervals." They are a basic concept in training, and they appear in various forms throughout the book.

Interval training simply means mixing work with recovery. In your case now, we're talking about jogging as being the "work" and walking as being the "recovery."

Because you aren't yet accustomed to jogging, the work periods are rather brief and the recovery time in between is long. As the month moves along, though, you'll do more jogging and less walking. You're moving toward a goal (which won't be reached until later in the book) of cutting out walking entirely.

Because you'll be working somewhat more intensively this month, I want you first of all to cut down your training time to a half-hour each day—nearly every day if possible.

Add the jogging on three of the days, with at least one day of only walking in between. For instance, you might walk-jog on Tuesday, Thursday and Saturday, and recover on the other days. (This is another application of the "interval" principle.)

This month, jog no more than a minute at a time, with no less than a minute's walk after each jog. In most towns, it takes about a minute to jog a block. Or you can go about a half-lap on a standard-sized track in that time. You can measure your jogs either of those ways. But the easiest and most exact method is to wear a wristwatch with a second hand and pace out your minute wherever you happen to be just then.

Don't race with yourself. I've warned against this before, and it's particularly risky now. You can't hurt yourself too much by walking too fast, but you can by running too fast. And it's tempting to try for speed in these first few weeks when you aren't ready to handle it.

Hold back. Jog slowly, with a relaxed, short, low stride. See that your breathing stays normal. Take spot checks of your pulse rate immediately after you finish a jog (put your hand over your heart, count the beats for six seconds and add a zero to the total). If it's higher than 150, slow down.

The goals for the month:

- Walk-jog on at least 12 days, and walk on at least 10 others —aiming for a total of a half-hour each day.
- Increase the total amount of jogging each week while decreasing the amount of walking.
- Keep the pulse rate below 150 beats per minute while jogging.
- Keep watching your resting pulse and weight, and keep reducing them if necessary.

# Third Month's Walking Plan

| Day | Suggested Training | Actual Training |
|---|---|---|
| 1 | 30-minute walk* | |
| 2 | extra exercise** | |
| 3 | 30-minute walk with one-minute jog*** | |
| 4 | extra exercise | |
| 5 | 30-minute walk with one-minute jog | |
| 6 | 30-minute walk | |
| 7 | 30-minute walk with 2 one-minute jogs | |
| *Weight at end of first week:*<br>*Resting pulse rate:* | | |
| 8 | extra exercise | |
| 9 | 30-minute walk | |
| 10 | 30-minute walk with 2 one-minute jogs | |
| 11 | extra exercise | |
| 12 | 30-minute walk with 2 one-minute jogs*** | |
| 13 | 30-minute walk | |

<table>
<tr><th>Day</th><th>Suggested Training</th><th>Actual Training</th></tr>
<tr><td>14</td><td>30-minute walk with<br>3 one-minute jogs</td><td></td></tr>
<tr><td colspan="3">Weight at end of second week:<br>Resting pulse rate:</td></tr>
<tr><td>15</td><td>extra exercise</td><td></td></tr>
<tr><td>16</td><td>30-minute walk</td><td></td></tr>
<tr><td>17</td><td>30-minute walk with<br>3 one-minute jogs</td><td></td></tr>
<tr><td>18</td><td>extra exercise</td><td></td></tr>
<tr><td>19</td><td>30-minute walk with<br>3 one-minute jogs</td><td></td></tr>
<tr><td>20</td><td>30-minute walk</td><td></td></tr>
<tr><td>21</td><td>30-minute walk with<br>4 one-minute jogs</td><td></td></tr>
<tr><td colspan="3">Weight at the end of third week:<br>Resting pulse rate:</td></tr>
<tr><td>22</td><td>extra exercise</td><td></td></tr>
<tr><td>23</td><td>30-minute walk</td><td></td></tr>
<tr><td>24</td><td>30-minute walk with<br>4 one-minute jogs</td><td></td></tr>
<tr><td>25</td><td>extra exercise</td><td></td></tr>
</table>

| Day | Suggested Training | Actual Training |
|---|---|---|
| 26 | 30-minute walk with 4 one-minute jogs | |
| 27 | 30-minute walk | |
| 28 | 30-minute walk with 5 one-minute jogs | |
| *Weight at end of fourth week:* *Resting pulse rate:* | | |
| 29 | makeup day**** | |
| 30 | makeup day | |
| 31 | makeup day | |

*Total number of walking-jogging days this month (20):* ________

*Net weight loss or gain for the month:* ____________________

*Net rise or fall in resting pulse rate:* ____________________

(*walk at a brisk and steady pace; **increasing the amount of normal daily activity—walking, bicycling, swimming, etc.—but not taking a formal workout; ***allow plenty of time to warm up by walking before attempting the one-minute jog, and recover for several minutes by walking between jogs and after the final one of the day; ****make up for sessions missed during the month)

# Lesson 8

# Questions

The first thing a Journalism I student is told on the first day of class is, "Answer the readers' questions right away—the five 'W's' and the 'H.' Those are: Who? What? When? Where? Why? How?"

Anyone who runs begins to feel like a journalist before he gets very far into the activity. That's because he's always being called upon to answer the same questions—particularly the last two. Non-runners want to know "Why?" New runners want to know "How?"

My job as a journalist and as a runner of some experience is to answer all the questions, with emphasis on the whys and hows. Each day's mail brings as many as a dozen letters asking for quick and simple answers. The phone brings a dozen more questions of the same type.

Most of the calls and letters come from people who are fairly new to running. I enjoy talking with them because the answers are so easy to give, and because the writers and callers are so grateful for any advice they receive.

The answers are easy to give because I respond to the same questions over and over again. They form a framework of information which new runners need as they start to build a program.

How, where and when do I run? How do I put a schedule together? What do I wear? These and several others are basic and recurring questions. I'll answer some of them here, and others as the book goes on.

- **How do I run?**

This is a question of form, of technique, of the way you move along the ground. The answer depends on the kind of moving you want to do, fast or slow. Sprinters don't run the same way as distance runners.

There are two guiding rules to running form:

The first is that form is largely an individual matter. It is a runner's "trademark," established by heredity and solidified by habit. Changes aren't easily made, and innocent quirks should be left alone. Concentrate on correcting form faults which result from blurry ideas of what running should be.

The second rule is that the faster you go, the more "up" and "out" you are. At top speed, you run on your toes and the stride is maximum length. At a jog, you land flat-footed or heel-first, and the stride is short.

The adjustment of foot plant and stride length to running speed occurs automatically if you let it. But the most common mistake slower runners make is trying to run like the milers or halfbacks they see on TV—with great, ground-gobbling strides,

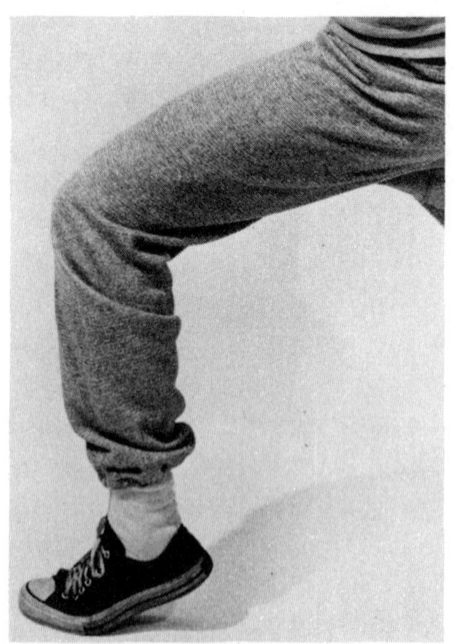

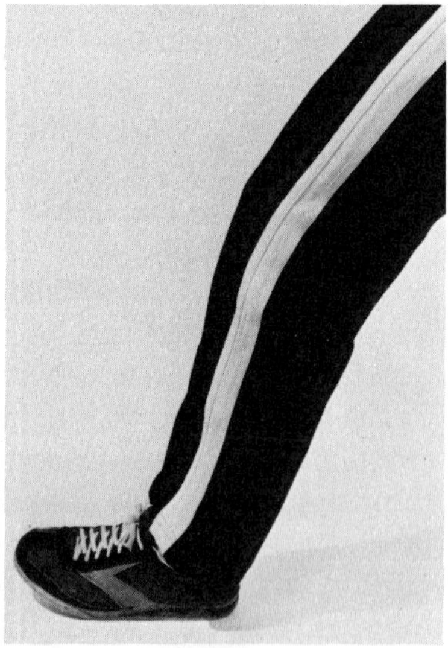

*The runner on the left lands too far up on the ball of his foot, while the other one uses the proper foot-plant for jogging.*

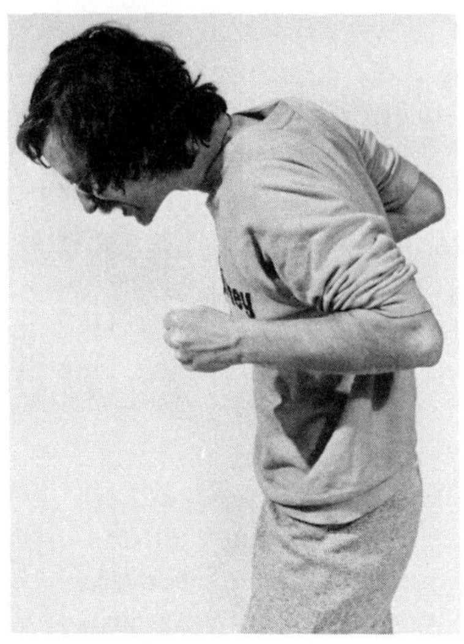

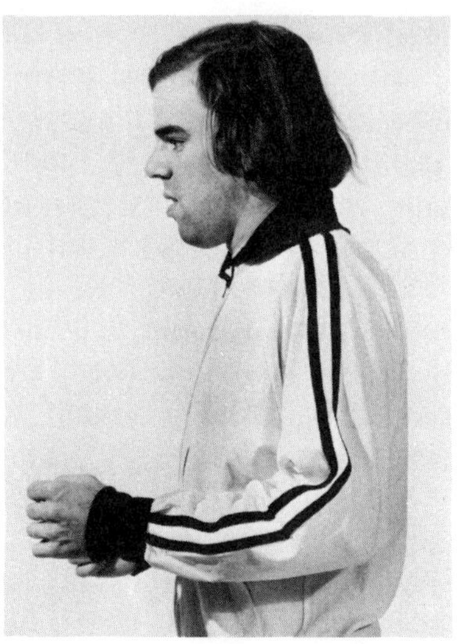

*Many beginners (left) run as if they're trying to punch down a wall. The ideal stance (right) is erect, with the arms relaxed.*

knees lifting too high, arms pumping too hard, heels never touching the surface, head bent forward like a battering ram.

If you're a distance runner, run like one. From the ground up, this involves:

*Feet*—It bears repeating that the slower you go the flatter you land, and vice versa.

*Stride*—Like foot-plant, this is a function of speed. Stride lengthens as you increase the pace, shortens as you slow. Don't overstride. Keep your feet under you. The point of foot contact should be directly under your knee, with the knee slightly flexed.

*Stance*—Run tall. Run with a straight back, the trunk directly over the legs. A distinct forward lean is helpful only if you're trying to batter down a wall with your head.

*Arms*—Don't lock the elbows. This creates tension and causes the shoulders to sway. Carry the arms in a position between the waistline and the bottom ribs, swinging them somewhat inward across the chest. Keep the hands loosely cupped.

*Head*—Look ahead, not at the sky or at your feet. This level-headed running insures that you run with an erect, balanced stance.

- **What do I wear?**

Good shoes and whatever else feels comfortable. Shoes are the first and most important investment a runner makes, because this is your only contact with the ground. Your health and performance rest on your feet, so protect them well. The rest of your clothing is just for warmth and decoration, so don't be as concerned about it.

Plan on spending $20-30 on shoes before you are very far into your running. There are several reasons for this. One obviously is protection, and you can't be sure of getting it for less than this price.

Canvas tennis sneakers won't do. They're too heavy and have too little support. Department and street shoe stores carry "running shoes" (actually cheap imitations of the standard brands) in the $10 range. Some are good, but you can't trust the quality. Some fall apart or wear down twice as fast as the more expensive models, so they're no bargain.

The final reason for buying good shoes is psychological. You *feel* more like a runner when you're shod like one. And you feel more of a commitment to continue if you've put $25 shoes on your feet.

Look for these features in your first shoes:

1. A soft, non-irritating upper of nylon or suede (or a combination of the two) to keep down the blister count.
2. Adequate room up front for your toes to spread out and not chafe.
3. Two-layer sole–a durable outer one which doesn't wear away like an eraser, and a soft and cushiony inner layer for shock absorption.
4. Heel which is about a half-inch higher than the sole. (This "lift" takes strain off the backs of the legs.)
5. Heel area supported and stabilized by a wide bottom of the shoe, a rigid "counter" or cup around the back and padding on the top rim.
6. A built-in arch support.

When you're trying on shoes, it's best to slip into a pair slightly on the large side rather than snug. This is because your feet tend to swell while running.

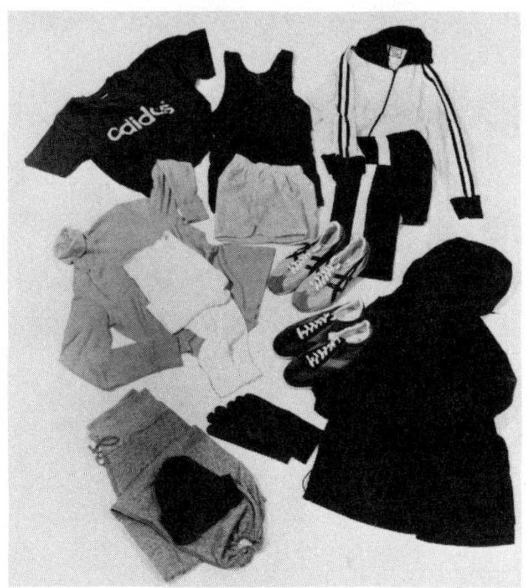


*Equipment for the well-dressed runner starts with shoes and shorts, and ends with a stocking cap, wind-breaker and gloves.*

You'll have no trouble finding good training flats. All of these are acceptable:

*Adidas* Runner, SL-72/76.

*Brooks* Trojan, Villanova.

*Eaton* Etonic.

*E.B. Sport International* Lydiard Road Runner.

*Karhu Models 2322, 2323.*

*New Balance* Models 220, 305, 320.

*Nike* Cortez, Road Runner, Waffle Trainer.

*Osaga* Moscow 80.

*Puma* Model 9190.

*Saucony* Hornet.

*Spotbilt* Model 850.

*Tiger* Grand Prix, Montreal 76.

As far as other clothing is concerned, there's no need to outfit yourself as if you were headed for the ski slopes. Some tips on dressing to run:

1. Keep the wardrobe simple and inexpensive. Use what you have available. Improvise instead of running up a clothing bill. (Save your money for shoes.) Loose-fitting, non-irritating shorts and long pants or shorts from the closet work for any purpose short of racing.

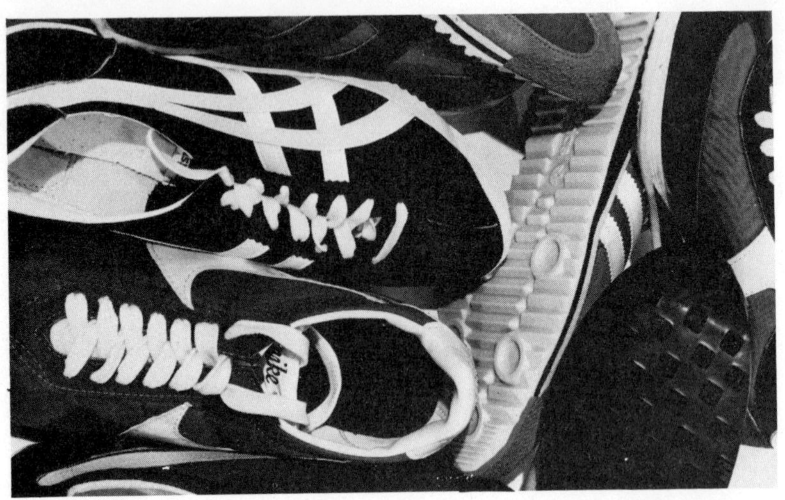

*In training flats, look primarily for a well-cushioned, flexible sole and an elevated, stable heel area. All the pictured shoes are adequate in these features.*

2. Dress inconspicuously. You'll feel better about running in public if your clothing doesn't attract special attention or show off bulges you want to hide.

3. Dress for the weather. In summer, wear as little as modesty allows. In winter, bundle up the head and hands. The arms, legs and trunk need little protection except on the coldest days. Don't overdress in any weather since you heat up quickly while running.

- **What do I do when the weather gets bad?**

First, define what you mean by "bad" and "good."

Is a bad day one on which a drizzle seems to be chilling you to the soul, one on which you work outside only reluctantly and then you must wear a jacket to stay warm?

Is a good day one which shines a warm sun on your bare shoulders and makes you wish you were stretched out at a pool or beach?

Not if you're planning to run. These days are defined this way by people who stand or lie still. For runners, they're just the opposite. The gray, drippy days are the good ones. The warm, sunny ones are not as nice as they look.

This is because the running body is its own furnace. It generates an astounding amount of heat as it exercises. And this heat warms you up well on cool to cold days, but it overheats you when the weather is warm to hot.

In short, the body is well equipped to warm itself during exercise. But it doesn't do so well at cooling itself off. For this reason, hot weather is a much bigger drain on a runner's energy and risk to his health than cold is. Yet we still tend to worry too much about the latter and ignore the former, staying inside in winter and going merrily out in the noonday sun in summer. Don't let first impressions of the seasons fool you.

What do you do when the weather goes to extremes? Keep running, by all means. If it's to do any good and to have any lasting value, you can't be a fair-weather runner. You have to keep going through good days and bad.

There will be some days which feel very bad. You can adjust your routine for them somewhat and make some adaptations, but you'll never avoid them completely. The adapting mostly takes care of itself. (As you run in the heat or cold, your body automatically resets its thermostat.) The adjustments are mostly common sense.

In hot weather, dress minimally, run at the coolest times of day (usually the temperature is lowest at dawn), drink all you can stand before and after running (maybe even during the run if it's a long one), and slow down or stop if you begin to feel dizzy or nauseated.

Sweat is the body's air-conditioning. It cools you as it evaporates. But high humidity messes up this cooling system because it slows evaporation. The body pumps out more sweat to compensate, but it never quite succeeds. This is why humid days always seem hotter than dry ones, though their temperature is the same.

Watch your weight closely in summer. Weigh in before and after running. If you're sweating away more than 3% of your body weight (five pounds or so), you're probably working too hard for the conditions. See that this liquid loss is replaced before you try to work hard again.

In cold weather, don't overdress (dress in layers so one or more can be peeled away as you run; the hands and ears need the most protection, the legs the least), run at the warmest hour of the day if possible (noon or early afternoon), don't stop during a run or stand around outside afterwards for long enough to get chilled, and run with the wind behind you when you can.

While it's humidity which makes summer days seem hotter, it's the wind which complicates winter running. Each mile per hour of headwind makes the air feel about one degree colder. So while the thermometer may read 20 above, a 20 m.p.h. wind can chill the effective temperature to below zero.

Regardless of temperature, however, there is no danger of "freezing your lungs." This is a mythical ailment widely feared by runners but never experienced by them or by the skiers and skaters they join outside in the cold.

The only real risks to winter runners are ice-coated surfaces and zero-visibility snowstorms. In these conditions, it is best to stay indoors.

## Heat Safety Index

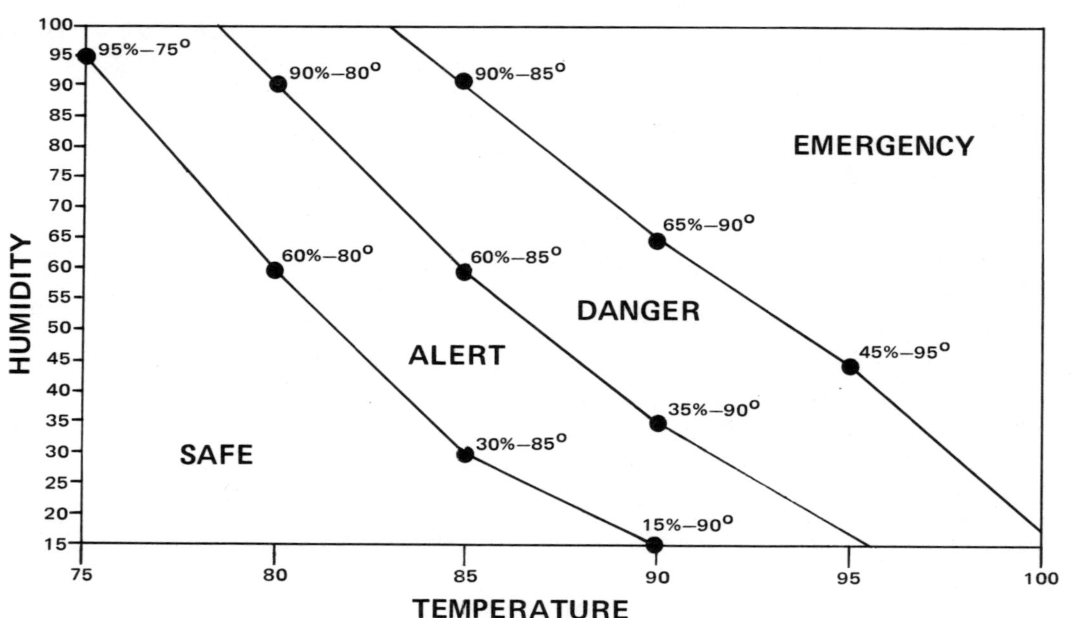


*The chart is adapted from the Weather Service Operations Manual. "Safe" temperature-humidity readings generally allow for normal activity. "Alert" conditions require caution during long, hard runs. "Danger" levels may demand a reduction of training. Strenuous running is not recommended during "emergency" conditions.*

# Wind-Chill Readings

| Wind (M.P.H.) | Temperature (Farenheit) | | | | | | | | | | | | | | | | | | | | |
|---|---|---|---|---|---|---|---|---|---|---|---|---|---|---|---|---|---|---|---|---|---|
| Calm | 40 | 35 | 30 | 25 | 20 | 15 | 10 | 5 | 0 | -5 | -10 | -15 | -20 | -25 | -30 | -35 | -40 | -45 | -50 | -55 | -60 |
| | Equivalent Chill Temperature | | | | | | | | | | | | | | | | | | | | |
| 5 | 35 | 30 | 25 | 20 | 15 | 10 | 5 | 0 | -5 | -10 | -15 | -20 | -25 | -30 | -35 | -40 | -45 | -50 | -55 | -65 | -70 |
| 10 | 30 | 20 | 15 | 10 | 5 | 0 | -10 | -15 | -20 | -25 | -35 | -40 | -45 | -50 | -60 | -65 | -70 | -75 | -80 | -90 | -95 |
| 15 | 25 | 15 | 10 | 0 | -5 | -10 | -20 | -25 | -30 | -40 | -45 | -50 | -60 | -65 | -70 | -80 | -85 | -90 | -100 | -105 | -110 |
| 20 | 20 | 10 | 5 | 0 | -10 | -15 | -25 | -30 | -35 | -45 | -50 | -60 | -65 | -75 | -80 | -85 | -95 | -100 | -110 | -115 | -120 |
| 25 | 15 | 10 | 0 | -5 | -15 | -20 | -30 | -35 | -45 | -50 | -60 | -65 | -75 | -80 | -90 | -95 | -105 | -110 | -120 | -125 | -135 |
| 30 | 10 | 5 | 0 | -10 | -20 | -25 | -30 | -40 | -50 | -55 | -65 | -70 | -80 | -85 | -95 | -100 | -105 | -115 | -120 | -130 | -140 |
| 35 | 10 | 5 | -5 | -10 | -20 | -25 | -35 | -40 | -50 | -60 | -65 | -75 | -80 | -90 | -100 | -105 | -115 | -120 | -130 | -135 | -145 |
| 40* | 10 | 0 | -5 | -15 | -20 | -30 | -35 | -45 | -55 | -60 | -70 | -75 | -85 | -95 | -100 | -110 | -115 | -125 | -130 | -140 | -150 |

**Little Danger**

**Increasing Danger** (Flesh may freeze within one minute)

**Great Danger** (Flesh may freeze within 30 seconds)

*Winds above 40 m.p.h. have little additional effect.

# PART THREE

# JOGGING

# Lesson 9

# Introducing Jogging

This is the season to be jogging. Three months from now, you can be jogging up to three miles and can be doing half that distance at good speed. And a nice thing about it will be that it won't take much time each day.

Jogging and running never need to take much time because they are fast-acting exercises. To draw the same physical benefits from a jog or run as you get from a walk, you need only about a fourth as much time. In other words, the effects of an hour's walk can be had in a 15-minute jog-run.

Before beginning the new season, perhaps it's worthwhile to make a couple of definitions:

The first is to define your own current level of fitness. If you haven't done so lately (or at all), take the fitness test in Lesson Four. You should have a score in the 10-19 range before starting to jog. If you're lower, back off to walking. If you're above 20, the jogging program may be too basic for you. Jump ahead to running (or at least to the second and third months of jogging, Lessons 13 and 15).

The second thing we need to define is jogging. What is a "jog," and how is it different from a "run"? Actually, a jog *is* a run—a *slow* run. How slow is "slow"? I could say seven minutes per mile, or eight, or 10. But I don't want to get involved in this kind of nitpicking or to make arbitrary divisions based on time.

As far as I'm concerned, the difference between jogging and running is not a matter of time but is a state of mind.

Jogging pace is a pace which *feels* comfortable—and one you can carry on without straining and puffing. For one person, seven minutes per mile might be jogging, while for another nine minutes might be hard running.

Jogging is also a matter of priorities. As I read their motivations, joggers are primarily interested in improving their physical fitness and doing so in a hurry. It's a perfectly legitimate and honorable ambition.

Runners, however, become so wrapped up in the activity for other reasons—usually recreation, relaxation or competition—that fitness becomes little more than a by-product.

You probably aren't fit enough yet to look beyond the goal of fitness, and to see the fun which lies on the other side. So stay with jogging for a while.

The three-month pattern here is similar to the one outlined earlier for walking, and is like the ones to be laid out later for running and racing. All that changes are the type of activity and the level of effort. At each stage, you're getting into something new. But it's nothing to fear because you have worked up to it gradually and are ready—eager, in fact—to handle a fresh challenge.

You either left off last month with a combination of walking and jogging, or your first fitness test said you could skip that phase and you're beginning here, with a combination of walking and jogging. Full-scale jogging will come in its own good time, and that time will be more rewarding if you save it for later rather than attempting to jog long or run fast before you have the fitness to do it.

Stay on schedule. Jump ahead of it *only* if it feels too easy for you. Judge the difficulty or ease not by how well you get through individual jogs, but by how fresh and eager you feel as the days and weeks add up.

- *First month*—This is the break-in period. At the start, more than half of each daily session still is walking. You're jogging in "intervals" of no more than a few minutes with longer walks in between. But as the month goes on, you shift from being primarily a walker to being a jogger. The jogs grow progressively longer while the walking total shrinks. By the month's end,

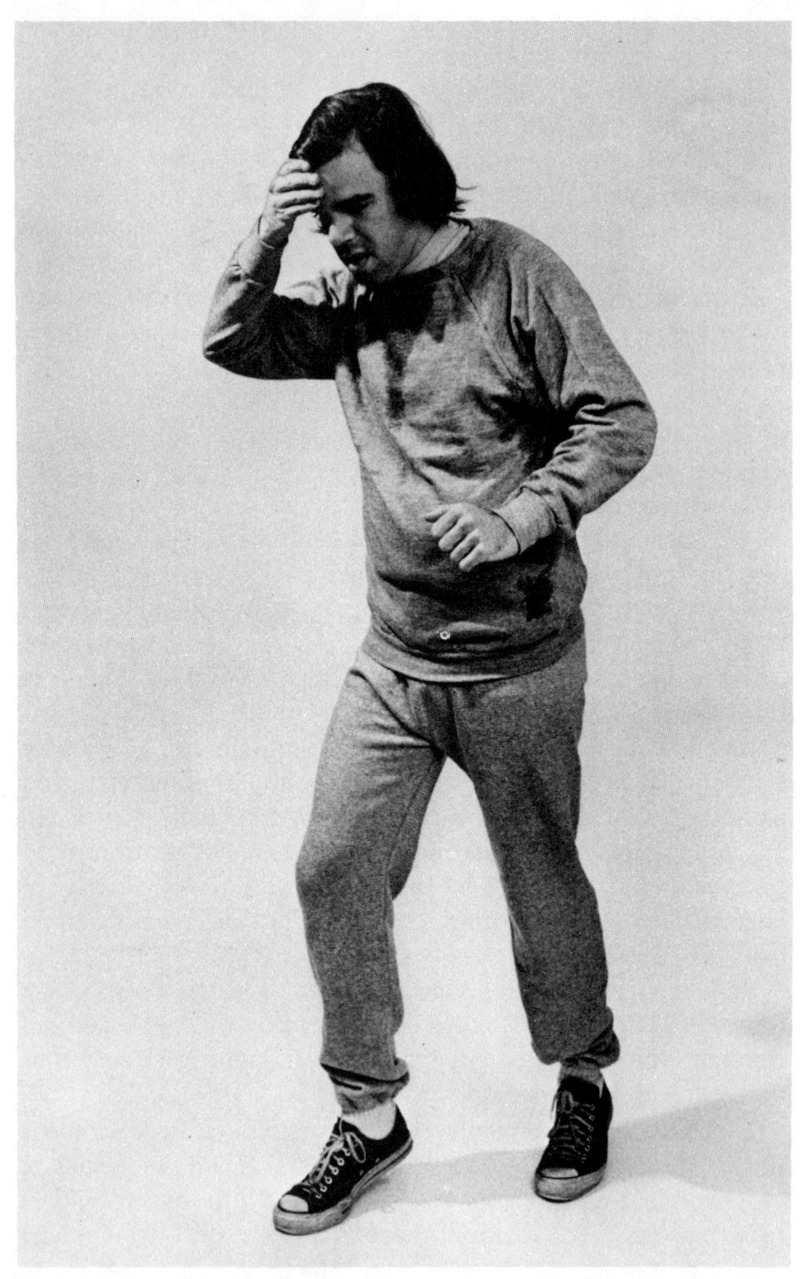

*"Joggers are primarily interested in improving their physical fitness and doing so in a hurry. It's a perfectly legitimate and honorable ambition . . . ."*

you're jogging continuously for a mile or 10-15 minutes.

• *Second month*–Pace isn't important yet. Distance is. This month, you're concentrating on building up the amount of gently-paced jogging. The goal is to double the longest jog of last month–to go between 20 and 30 minutes or 2-3 miles in one stretch–and to *average* the 10-15 minutes which recently had been a peak effort.

• *Third month*–This is the month for speeding up. You are jogging far enough for now and are ready to do it a little faster. I don't mean that you're free to time your distances every day and to work at improving the times daily. This is racing, and you are not ready for it.

What you are ready to do is introduce some running. Introduce it in the same way the walkers began to jog in earlier lessons–little by little. Add short "intervals" of faster running, so you can get used to the feeling of speed without experiencing the exhaustion which can go with it.

At the end of the month, you take your first timed test, seeing how much distance you can cover in 12 minutes. This is a standard test taken by millions of people, and your results may surprise you.

# Lesson 10

# Talk Like A Runner

Normally, he's one of your best friends. In other situations, you are equals. But now you resent him for his air of superiority. You resent the paternal attitude he has taken toward you since you announced, "I want to start doing a little jogging. Can you give me some pointers?"

He's done a lot more than give pointers. Once you gave him this small opening, he rushed in and has almost smothered you with printed and verbal advice and encouragement. He has met you at the local high school track every morning to help you through your run. You resent your childlike dependence on him, but you both know you need him.

Your friend is a serious runner, a racer. He has the hollow-cheeked, hungry look common to men in his sport. He's the type no one would ever pick from a crowd to call "athlete." Yet you're now coming to appreciate how much athletic talent is concealed within that skinny frame.

He runs his five or 10 or 15 miles, then comes to the track and runs with you during his "warmdown"–whatever that means. His 15th mile is easier for him than your first is for you. You resent him for the way he can jabber along while you struggle for the breath to gasp "yup" and "nope."

Today, as you're finishing your mile, your friend sees another runner across the track and shouts a greeting. The other man bounds over to you with disgusting energy. He has the same hollow cheeks and sinewy body as your friend. There are introductions, then the two of them get to talking.

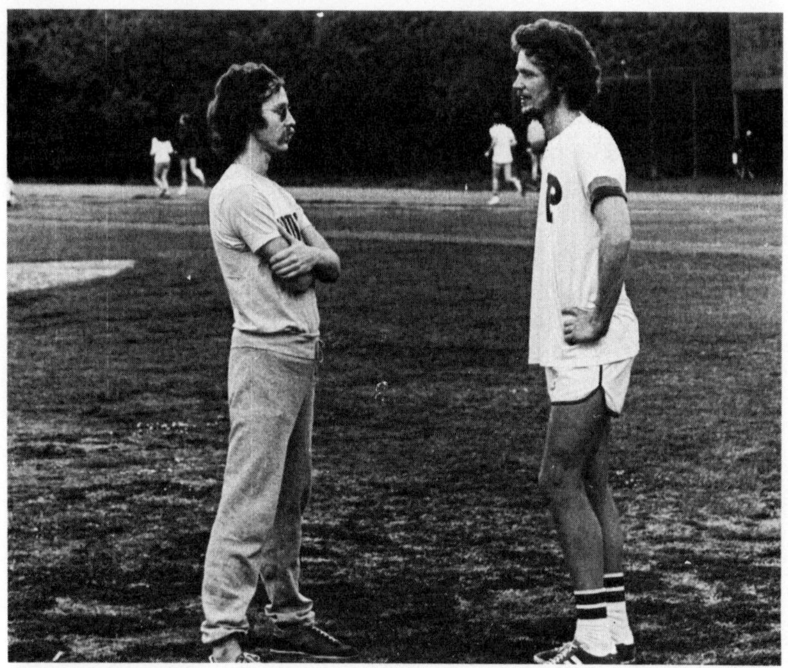

*"Every specialty has its own working language in order to avoid wasting words. These code words say a lot with a little breath . . . ."*

"What've you been up to since I saw you last?"

"No much. Had a stress fracture of the metatarsals, then chondromalacia from overcompensating. The podiatrist told me I had Morton's Foot, and he gave me orthotics. What's happening with you?"

"I've been doing some sharpening for the middle distances. That's why I'm here at the track today, to do some speed work. It's a crash program of quarter intervals at 65 pace with a 220 recovery. Have you been racing?"

"Not for a while. But I have an ultra-marathon this weekend –a 50-K. I'm tapering for it now–just doing short jogs, a few pickups and some stretching. Tell me about the middle distances you're doing."

"I raced a mile last week. It wasn't so good. 4:55. I went out too fast and got into oxygen debt. The bear jumped on my back in the third quarter. Rig set in so bad I was crawling the rest of the way. I had no kick at all."

"Maybe you should forget this short stuff and get back to LSD."

"I think I will. It's about time to start getting ready for Boston. Say, are you loading for the race this weekend?"

"Oh, sure. I took my depletion run last Saturday. I'm through with the protein phase now and am ready to start stuffing the carbos."

"I've gotta run. See you."

Your friend waves at the disappearing runner, and you stand staring at him with your mouth hanging open. You haven't understood a thing the two of them have said. You resent them for speaking a language which excludes you. It's a language for insiders which assures you that you're still very much an outsider in this activity.

Every specialty has its own working language in order to avoid wasting words on the job. These code words say a lot with a little breath. The sooner you start slipping these words into your speech, the sooner you'll slip into the inner circle of runners. Toward that end, here is a beginning runner's dictionary:

### –A–

*AAU*–short for Amateur Athletic Union, the group which controls much of the running competition in the United States and certifies runners' eligibility to race.

*Achilles*–a long, thin tendon connecting the heel bone with the calf muscle in the back of the leg; source of a high percentage of runners' injuries.

*Addiction*–the condition runners claim they achieve after a few months to a few years in the activity; once you reach the point where it feels worse not to run that to do it, you're addicted; a positive goal.

*Aerobic*–with a small "a," it means "with oxygen;" its opposite is *an*aerobic (without oxygen); more commonly, it's called Aerobics with a capital "A," referring to the exercise program established by Dr. Kenneth Cooper; recommended activities (jogging, walking, bicycling, etc.) supply strong, steady oxygen doses.

*Age-group*–competition often is separated by age; major

groupings are "junior" (19 and under), "open" (20-39) and "Master" (40 and up); among Masters, there are further breakdowns into 10- and five-year groups, and juniors have even finer divisions; records are kept for each year of age on all levels.

*All-comers*—running events open to everyone, regardless of age, affiliation or ability.

*All-weather track*—the kind you love when it rains; surface is a rubber-asphalt mixture or artificial material; often lumped under the name "Tartan," though that is only one brand of track.

**—B—**

*Base*—the ability to run for a long time without tiring; built by running for a long time at a non-tiring level of effort.

*Bear*—a figurative creature who jumps on your back and drags you down when you've run too far, too fast or a combination of the two.

*Belly-breathing*—deep breathing which causes the abdomen to swell and protrude on inhaling; helpful both in taking in enough air and in the elimination of sideaches called "stitches."

*Biathlon*—this competitive event combines swimming and distance running, two complementary aerobic activities.

*Boston*—THE long-distance race in the United States; classic marathon (26 miles 385 yards) which has gone on since the 1890s.

*Burst*—a sudden increase in speed during a run or race, usually carried on for only a short distance; used as a training variation or a tactical tool.

**—C—**

*Carbohydrate-loading*—a diet-juggling technique to increase staying power in a long race; includes eating mainly high-energy starchy and sugary foods during the last three days before an event.

*Cardiovascular*—pertaining to the heart and the blood vessels; a main benefit of jogging and running is in tuning up and strengthening this system.

*Certified*—a racing course which is guaranteed accurate in distance; measured according to precise methods set up by the ruling bodies of the sport.

*Chondromalacia*—also known as "runner's knee" because it strikes people in this activity so often; a wear-and-tear injury causing cramping pain around the kneecap.

*Collapse point*—the point where "the bear" jumps on, where "rig" sets in, where you can go no farther; in terms of distance, this point often is reached at about three times your daily average mileage.

*Cooper*—Dr. Kenneth Cooper, the developer of the Aerobics system, author of several books on the subject and one of the most influential men in the running-for-fitness movement.

*Cross-country*—running on "natural" terrain—grass, dirt, beach, etc.; the season for cross-country racing in the United States is autumn, September through November.

**–D–**

*Depletion run*—the final long and/or hard run before a big race; usually done about a week in advance, as part of the carbohydrate-loading routine.

*DNF*—an aborted run; the letters stand for "did not finish."

**–E–**

*Electrolytes*—the minerals in the foods you eat and liquids you drink; potassium, magnesium and sodium are the most important to runners because these minerals are sweated away quickly.

*Endurance*—staying power; the ability to run long distances; depends on the efficiency of the heart and circulatory system, and on how well you take in and use oxygen.

*Exercise physiology*—the study of the inner workings of the body during activity; the scientists who do the studying are physiologists.

**–F–**

*Fartlek*—this strange-sounding word is Swedish for "speed play"; it describes a training method involving free-form changes of pace.

*Fast distance*—steady-paced training runs, usually timed and over known distances, and close to one's maximum effort.

*Fitness*—not a synonym for "health"; health implies a mere absense of disease; fitness is the ability to put one's health to work in a positive, dynamic way.

*Flats*—running shoes designed for roads and cross-country courses; they come in sturdy styles for training and lighter ones for racing.

*Flexibility*—running tends to make the leg muscles stiff and tense, yet their ability to move freely (flexibly) is a criteria of fitness; supplemental flexibility exercises are recommended to all runners.

*Form*—the way a runner moves; also known as "style" or "technique."

*Fun-running*—the school of thinking which emphasizes neither physical fitness nor serious competition, but running for the enjoyment of it; some informal races also go by the name of Fun-Runs.

**—H—**

*Half*—a short way of saying "half-mile," which is 880 yards.

*Hard-easy*—this theory of training holds that after each hard effort there must be adequate recovery; recommended is one or two easy days of running after each hard one.

*Heat exhaustion and stroke*—the most serious threats to a runner's health and life; these medical conditions are caused by running too long or hard in hot, humid weather; they require immediate professional treatment.

**—I—**

*Indoor*—indoor track running on tracks rarely less than eight laps per mile; the indoor racing season in the United States lasts from December through March.

*Intervals*—training which alternates rather short and fast runs with periods of jogging, walking or rest; a typical workout is 10 fast 440s with a 440-yard recovery jog-walk after each.

**—J—**

*Jog*—there is no way to define it more precisely than to say it is a slow run; perhaps a better way to separate jogging from running (if indeed a separation is needed) is to say that jogging is done primarily for physical exercise while running is more for recreation and competition.

*Junior*—an age category in racing taking in runners 19 and younger.

**—K—**

*K*—abbreviated version of kilometer (see below), as in a 10-K race.

*Kick*—the increase in speed at the end of a run or race.

*Kilometer*—a basic unit of measurement in the metric system; 1000 meters is equal to about 1100 yards or five-eighths of a mile; almost all distance races now are run in kilometers—five, 10, 15, 20, 25, 30 and 50 being the standard ones.

**—L—**

*Lactic acid*—a chemical substance in the blood which results from severe effort and leads to muscle fatigue; a cause of "the bear" or "hitting the wall."

*Long distances*—in practice, anything farther than you normally go seems long; in racing, the long distances generally are defined as those beyond 10,000 meters; usually run on the roads.

*LSD*—the initials stand for "long, slow distance"; a way of training which emphasizes lots of steady running at moderate effort.

*Lydiard*—Arthur Lydiard, a pioneering coach from New Zealand whose methods in training both joggers and racers are widely copied.

**—M—**

*Marathon*—a word widely misused to apply to any endurance contest; in running, it only means the classic race of 26 miles 385 yards (42.195 kilometers).

*Masters*—the branch of age-group competition limited to men 40 and over, and women 30 and up; also called "seniors" and "veterans."

*Metatarsals*—small bones in the forefoot which frequently are damaged in running.

*Middle distances*—races in the half-mile to six-mile (800-10,000-meter) range, usually run on the track.

*Morton's Foot*—an inborn condition most easily recognized by the second toe being longer than the big toe; runners with this type of feet are thought to be highly susceptible to foot and lower-leg injuries.

## –O–

*Open*—competition in which anyone and everyone is eligible to race; most road races are unrestricted.

*Overcompensation injuries*—"sympathetic pains" caused by favoring a sore spot in another part of the body—usually the opposite leg in runners.

*Overdistance*—training runs beyond the usual racing distance or longer than the daily average.

*Overuse*—a fancy word for working too hard before you are ready; most running injuries occur this way, from wear and tear rather than by accident.

*Oxygen debt*—needing more air than you can take in; you're in debt when your breathing is labored during a run; the debt is repaid when you slow down or stop.

*Oxygen uptake*—a measurement of the amount of oxygen the body processes during exercise; an excellent indication of endurance fitness.

## –P–

*Pace*—the average rate of running, expressed in such terms as "70-second quarters" or "five-minute miles"; pacing yourself means spreading your effort evenly over the entire distance of the run.

*Pickups*—increases in pace for short distances during longer runs; used as training or tactics.

*Podiatrist*—a doctor who specializes in treatment of the feet and lower legs; one of the best friends a sore runner can have.

*PR*—the initials represent "personal record" times, the most significant marks a runner can set; this is one of the few sports which allows you to measure yourself against your former self.

*Preventive medicine*—health practices which operate on the

principle that it is easier to stay well than to get well, easier to prevent than to treat.

*Pulled muscle*—actually all muscles "pull" during exercise; this is their normal function; the injury which goes by this name is a tear in the muscle fibers.

**—Q—**

*Quality*—training which is rather short and intensive as opposed to long and leisurely.

*Quarter*—short for quarter-mile, the length of one lap on the standard outdoor track.

**—R—**

*Race walking*—more than a gentle stroll; this is competitive walking, at paces which rival those of slow running; the training, competitive practices and physical-psychological benefits of this sport are much the same as in running.

*Resistance work*—training up hills, through loose dirt or sand, or with extra weight on the feet or upper body; anything which causes more than the usual amount of "drag" while running.

*Rig*—short for "rigor mortis," which is what you feel is setting in when you approach exhaustion.

*RRC*—Road Runners Club, an international organization with local branches in the US which promote long-distance competition.

*Running*—an all-inclusive term covering everything above a walk; jogging, sprinting, racing all are forms or degrees of running.

**—S—**

*Sanction*—official approval for one of the sport's governing bodies to conduct a race; most US distance races are sanctioned by the AAU and RRC.

*Sciatica*—inflammation in one of the longest nerves in the body; sciatic nerve runs from the lower back down the back of each leg to the foot; source of frequent injuries in runners.

*Senior*—confusing word because it is defined in many ways: "senior" in high school or college; "senior" competition in the AAU, which is synonymous with "open," all-age racing; or "senior" as meaning the same as "Master" (age 40 and up); if you want to be clear in what you're saying, use another word.

*Sharpening*—training to gain an edge in speed; usually comes after a "base" in endurance has been laid down.

*Shin splints*—one of the most common running injuries, particularly with beginners; pain and tenderness along the bone in the front of the lower leg.

*Short distances*—another name for the sprints; runs of 440 yards-400 meters and less.

*Speed*—strictly speaking, speed is an absolute—the fastest one's born-in and trained-in abilities will allow him to go; also called "basic speed" or "raw speed."

*Spikes*—the shoes worn for racing on the track; light in construction and equipped with 4-7 sharp spikes.

*Splits*—times given for a portion of the full distance; for instance, quarter-mile times at one, two and three laps en route to a mile.

*Sports medicine*—while conventional medicine stresses the treatment of disease and preservation of health, sports medicine operates on a higher plane; it emphasizes gaining and maintaining fitness for maximum performances.

*Sprints*—the races in which the paces are all-out all the way; distances of 400 yards-400 meters and less.

*Stamina*—differs subtly from the definition of endurance; endurance is the ability to hold any effort for a long time; runners talk of stamina in terms of being able to hold a high level of effort for the full distance of the run.

*Steady state*—the dividing line between aerobic (normal breathing) and anaerobic (out-of-breath) running; as fitness increases, the pace at which you can run in a "steady state" grows faster.

*Stitch*—a sharp pain in the side, occurring while running; usually related to faulty breathing, diet or running form.

*Strength*—a term often confused with endurance or stamina; actually, strength is the ability to make heavy, explosive efforts, such as lifting a weight.

*Stress*—both a necessity and a curse for runners; stress simply is any hardship, physical or mental; a certain amount must be applied or a runner never improves, but with too much he breaks down; training is a process of applying the right kind and quality of stress.

*Stress fracture*—a hairline break in a bone, usually one of the tiny foot bones or in the shin; it generally occurs from the stress of running rather than an accident.

*Stress test*—an evaluation of the heart's capacity for work, made while you work at a level approximating that of running; recommended for all beginners in their 30s and older.

*Stretching*—exercises to loosen the muscles which grow tight and inflexible during running; used to prevent soreness and injuries.

*Style*—another word for the way you look when you run; also called "form" or "technique."

*Survival shuffle*—the way runners continue to struggle ahead toward the finish line after they've gone farther and faster than was wise.

*Sweats*—clothing runners wear for cold weather and/or for warming up; long pants and long-sleeved shirt or jacket.

**–T–**

*Tactics*—tricks used in racing to gain steps on an opponent; necessary only if you consider beating someone to be important.

*Talk test*—a key check of whether or not the training pace is right for building endurance; if you can talk, whistle or sing normally, you aren't going too fast.

*Tapering*—cutting back on the amount of running being done in order to gather energy for a big effort; racers taper from a day to a week or more before a big race.

*Tartan*—the Cadillac of the all-weather tracks; made of a bouncy artificial material.

*Tendonitis*—inflammation of the connective cords called tendons; runners most often suffer in the lateral (sides of feet), achilles (heel) and knee tendons.

*Time trial*—a simulated race, timed, over a known distance and at racing effort, but usually done alone.

*Training*—in the strict sense, it means preparing now for some future reward; many runners who say their rewards are immediate do not use this term.

*Training effect*—a combined term for the variety of physical and mental changes which indicate that you are adapting to the stress of running.

**—U—**

*Ultra-distances*—also called "ultra-marathons"; races longer than the marathon distance of 26.22 miles.

*Underdistance*—training runs shorter than the usual distance; usually run as fast as racing pace or faster.

**—V—**

*Van Aaken*—Europe's answer to American running-for-fitness advocate Dr. Kenneth Cooper; Dr. Ernst van Aaken of West Germany has built his method around long endurance runs mixed with very small amounts of faster running.

*Veteran*—the European equivalent of the US "Master"; runners age 40 and up.

**—W—**

*Wall*—the invisible yet real barrier a runner hits when he's exhausted by the distance or pace of a run.

*Warmup and warmdown*—pre- and post-run activities to get the body revved up and cooled down; combinations of exercises, walking, jogging and faster striding.

*Weight training*—lifting barbells and dumbells to increase strength and correct muscular imbalances; most helpful to sprinters who rely on explosive muscular power.

**—Y—**

*Yoga*—gentle, slow-motion stretching exercises which have been found to be ideal in correcting the muscle tightness common to runners.

The words won't do any good with non-runners. You'll confuse and bore them now and later with talk of running. So save the words for people already in the activity-sport. They're starved for conversation on their favorite subject, so they'll be happy to hear someone new who's trying to speak their language.

Don't pretend to know everything. Otherwise, you'll end up

like you do when you say "Buenos dias" to a Mexican cab driver. You'll turn loose a torrent of unfamiliar words. Try out your new language carefully. When a runner asks, "How's it going for you?" you might answer this way:

"Slowly. The first mile is the hardest, they tell me, so I guess I'm still in the hardest part. I'm following the Aerobics program—jogging every other day, and supplementing that with the equivalent amount of walking or bicycling on the other days.

"I'm making sure I can pass the talk test when I jog, so right now I almost have to walk to go slow enough to breathe normally."

Before you know it, he's offering you unsolicited but much-needed encouragement and advice because you know enough words to sound interested—but not so many that you sound wise.

# Lesson 11

# Break In

This is the month you put much of your walking behind you. If you had to start with walking, be happy you used it. It laid the foundation on which jogging can be built. But walking is not a substitute for jogging and running. They are different actions with different effects.

If you want to be a jogger/runner, you don't get that way by walking, any more than you become a swimmer by taking frequent baths. Those baths may overcome a fear of getting wet, but they don't hone the swimming strokes. The walks get you used to moving again and harden the leg muscles, but they don't perfect running technique.

You're moving beyond walking now. And as this month goes along, it gradually will shrink out of your training. Walking still is fine recreation and transportation, and I urge you to keep using it that way every chance you get. But start turning over most of the training time to the activities this book is written to promote.

Walking's role shifts from a primary to a supplementary one. It now supports jogging instead of preparing you for it as it had in the earlier lessons.

Walk to warm up for a day's jogging. The muscles–including the most important muscle, the heart–aren't ready to go directly from rest to a brisk jog. (This is particularly true early in the morning.) They may rebel. So walk for several minutes before breaking into a jog.

By the same token, it's wise to walk for several more minutes at the end of a session so the transition from jogging to rest won't be too abrupt. The purpose is to cool off a bit before stopping, but for some reason it is called a "warmdown" instead of a "cooldown."

Walking also continues to have a role in recovery. For now, you'll be breaking many jogs into several segments, with walks between, to let you go farther without exhausting yourself. And by doing more walking on your "easy" days, you're fresher to do more jogging on the "hard" days.

There are three of these hard days a week. But don't take that word too seriously. They are hard only in the sense that they are "building" days and the others are for recovery. Alternate the easy with the hard.

Starting this month, make one of the days–preferably a Saturday or Sunday–a Big One. This is a day for pushing ahead into territory you haven't explored before. Go up to twice as far as you are accustomed to jogging. If, for instance, you're averaging five non-stop minutes per day during the week, jog up to 10 minutes on Saturday.

The main goal for the month is to jog continuously for 10-15 minutes or to cover one mile. Go either by time or distance, but don't attempt to time yourself for a measured distance. Speed doesn't count yet.

A second goal is to increase the total amount of jogging you do each week.

Third, do some jogging at least 20 days of the month, and at least take informal walks on most other days.

Fourth, keep trying to reduce your weight and resting pulse toward your ideals.

Fifth, keep your exercise pulse rate below 150 (spot-check yourself to see how fast your heart is beating by counting beats for six seconds as you stop jogging. Add a zero to the total.)

# First Month's Jogging Plan

| Day | Suggested Training | Actual Training |
|---|---|---|
| 1 | 3-minute jog* | |
| 2 | rest** | |
| 3 | 3 one-minute jogs | |
| 4 | 3-minute jog | |
| 5 | rest | |
| 6 | 3 one-minute jogs | |
| 7 | 5-minute jog | |
| *Week's total of jogging (17 minutes):* | | |
| 8 | rest | |
| 9 | 3 one-minute jogs | |
| 10 | 5-minute jog | |
| 11 | rest | |
| 12 | 5-minute jog | |
| 13 | 3 one-minute jogs | |
| 14 | 8-minute jog | |
| *Week's total of jogging (24 minutes):* | | |

| Day | Suggested Training | Actual Training |
|---|---|---|
| 15 | rest | |
| 16 | 3 one-minute jogs | |
| 17 | 8-minute jog | |
| 18 | rest | |
| 19 | 8-minute jog | |
| 20 | 3 one-minute jogs | |
| 21 | 10-minute jog | |
| *Week's total of jogging (32 minutes):* | | |
| 22 | rest | |
| 23 | 3 one-minute jogs | |
| 24 | 10-minute jog | |
| 25 | rest | |
| 26 | 10-minute jog | |
| 27 | 3 one-minute jogs | |
| 28 | 15-minute jog | |
| *Week's total of jogging (41 minutes):* | | |

| Day | Suggested Training | Actual Training |
|---|---|---|
| 29 | makeup day*** | |
| 30 | makeup day | |
| 31 | makeup day | |

*Total number of training days for month (20):*____________

*Total amount of jogging for month (114 minutes):*__________

*Average jogging amount per day (5.7 minutes):*____________

*Weight at beginning and end of month:* _________________

*Resting pulse rate at beginning and end of month:*__________

(*all jogging this month is included in a total workout of 20-30 minutes, with the remainder of the time taken up by walking as warmup and recovery; ** "rest" days should include some physical activity—walking, bicycling, swimming, etc.; ***make up for sessions missed during the month)

## Lesson 12

# Learn the Laws

A runner is a runner is a runner. And putting him into one of the subdivisions of that category doesn't change what he is.

He may be a racer or a jogger, a sprinter or a hurdler, a speedster or a slogger, a male or a female, a Junior or a Master. His main purpose in running may be fun or fellowship, competition or conditioning, solitude or speed, testing or therapy. There is room under the title "runner" for all types and aims.

All degrees and descriptions of runners are alike in more ways than they're different. They all operate under the same physical laws. They all get more from running if they work within those laws, and they all suffer when they break them.

A beginner runs the same way as an Olympic champion. Not so fast and so far, of course. Not with the same power, grace and single-minded fury. But they have the same principles guiding them.

Learn the laws, and the specifics of day-to-day running will write themselves.

- **Be specific.**

You pick what you plant. Just as you can't expect to put potatoes into the ground and harvest tomatoes, you can't become a runner by bowling or lifting weights.

There is little, if any, carry-over benefit from other activities—even the closely related ones like walking, swimming and bicycling. You learn to run by running. And so your running time is most profitably spent in doing just that.

This law applies even more specifically within running. You

learn the type of running you practice, so it should relate closely in distance and pace to your main purpose. If you're a sprinter, sprint. If you're a distance runner, run long distances.

- **Stress the positive.**

Stress is not a horrible force bent on wrecking our lives, something to be avoided at all costs. Stress is an important part of living, with a positive as well as a negative side.

Stress is like a series of waves crashing against the shoreline. We can react against it in one of two ways. We can surrender to it and let it wash us away. Or we can react by building walls which would have stayed weak without the pressure from stress.

Running is a stress. When it's applied in small doses, the body reacts by strengthening its defenses against this and other stresses. Runners require specific and regular stresses in order to adapt and improve.

- **Form a habit.**

Become "addicted." That's the easiest way to insure improvement in running. Longtime runners say that it took them a few months to form a running habit. After that, it took more effort *not* to run than to do it. Running became as much a part of each day as getting up and going to bed.

Getting hooked this way insures the continuity needed in any good running program. The benefits of running pile up quickly, but the reverse is also true. They vanish during a few weeks off. To keep the gains ahead of the losses, plan to run at least three days each week, the year round.

- **Take a break.**

The running puzzle has two parts, and one is no good without the other. The two are work and rest. You can't go anywhere unless you work. But you can't work hard all the time. Rest must follow work as surely as a night's sleep follows a day's activity.

This is the "interval principle" which is basic to all running. It insists on recurring cycles of work and recovery within individual runs, through the week, and over longer periods of months, seasons and years.

Run when you're eager, rest when you're tired, and learn to

tell the two feelings apart. Knowing when to stop is as important as knowing how to start.

- **Shift the load.**

Rare is the runner who recovers well enough from a hard run to take the same run again the next day, and the day after that, and again the following days.

Running energies rarely flow that smoothly or come back that quickly. Even if physical recovery happens that way, seldom does the mind thrive on a same-thing-every-day schedule.

Runners seem to stay fresher and more eager, and to improve quicker, on "hard-easy" or "long-short" routines. This means never running hard two days in a row. It's a variation of the "interval" theme in the previous law.

This may translate to hard runs three days a week, easy ones on the other days for an experienced athlete. A beginner who feels that any run is hard might run one day and rest the next.

- **Pace yourself.**

Run at a rate which will take you the whole distance you plan to go. This advice is obvious when you're thinking of a single run. If you're going three miles, you don't start at sprint pace. Otherwise, you won't finish.

What isn't so obvious is the long-term application of the pacing concept. If you plan to keep running for years, you can't burn yourself out in the first few weeks. Otherwise, you won't get to next month.

Pace yourself for the distance you want to go.

- **Learn to endure.**

Endurance comes first. Before you can go anywhere in this sport, you have to develop the power to last the distance. You must build a base.

You can't run hard and fast until you can run easy and slow. Always be sure you can run a distance easily before you think about racing it.

Never attempt to run a distance at any pace if it is beyond your trained-in capacity. That limit called the "collapse point," is generally thought to be about three times your average daily distance.

• **Approach speed cautiously.**

Speed running is necessary only if you race. But for racers, it is essential. It also is risky.

Speed does no good unless it's built on top of a solid foundation of endurance. Yet it's true, too, that endurance can't be used in a race until speed training is added to it.

Speedwork is the racer's edge. But it must be approached with caution because in it hide injuries and exhaustion. A wise runner doesn't let it take up more than a small percentage of his training time. Fortunately, he doesn't need more than a small dose. Speed comes quickly, while endurance develops slowly but lasts longer.

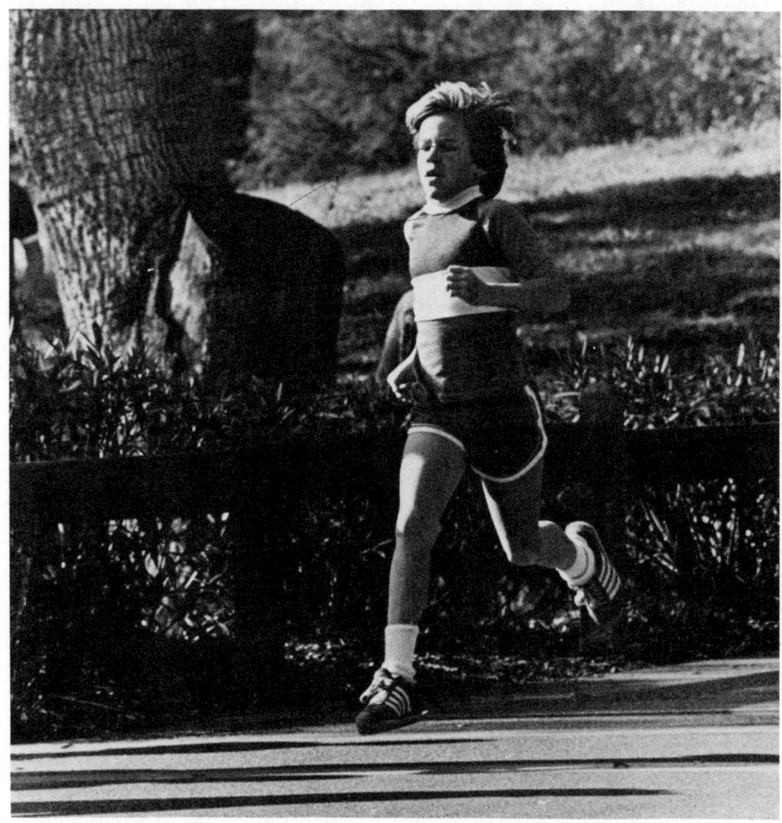

*Older runners re-learn many of the laws which children know instinctively. Much wisdom comes from watching how the young run.*

- **See progress.**

The big advantage of running over most other sports and fitness activities is that its results are so easily measured. And those measurements are both objective and personal. You can see clearly where *you* are going.

While measuring progress, keep a couple of facts in mind:

1. Improvement doesn't come in direct proportion to the work invested. You probably get 90% of the benefits from running in the first mile or two. And to tap each percentage point of your potential after that, you must put in an increasing amount of effort. In other words, each new mile gives you less than the one before. This is the law of diminishing returns at work.

2. The same law is at work when you first become a runner. You'll make the most progress from the least miles in the first weeks. Then as you approach the condition you want to be in, progress will be slower in coming.

- **Set and reach goals.**

It's as important to reach them as to set them. Aiming for the stars is fine, but you get discouraged in a hurry if you never touch them. Keep your stars within reach. Set goals which are realistic, which are a few inches beyond your fingertips. Then as they're reached, set slightly higher ones.

Every runner needs goals so he'll keep striving. But luckily, goals in running are easily and personally set because of its combination of distances and times. You only need to measure yourself against the odometer, the stop watch and your former self.

# Lesson 13

# Build Up

As you progress upward in fitness, an encouraging thing happens. Work which a few weeks ago had been exhausting, if not impossible, becomes routine. It's a heady feeling, for example, to jog a mile for recovery on an "easy" day, while just a month ago this had been the outer limit of your fitness.

The first mile is the hardest one to jog. It takes a while to break out of your resting inertia. But once you've overcome that first mile, the next few come easier. This month, you'll nearly double your amount of jogging, and yet you won't be suffering for this increase. It won't hurt as much as last month did, because you're ready now to move up quickly. You have laid the foundation by walking and jogging, and if you've come this far you're eager to see how much farther you can go.

You're moving into a program of the type runners use. It is a blend of short, medium and long sessions. A typical week of training might be put together in this pattern:

*Sunday*—rest or walk only; no jogging.

*Monday*—short-easy day; jog about half your average distance or time. For instance, you may total 75 minutes for the week, in five jogs. The daily average is 15 minutes. Jog 7-8 minutes on short days.

*Tuesday*—medium-hard day; jog your average distance or time.

*Wednesday*—rest or walk only; no jogging.

*Thursday*—medium-hard day; jog your average distance or time.

*Friday*—short-easy day; jog about half your average distance or time.

*Saturday*—long-hard day; jog 1½-2 times your average. If the average is 15 minutes, go 22-30 this day. Perhaps slow down the pace and take a few short walking breaks so you can finish without undue strain.

The intent this month is to increase rather quickly your total jogging time (and therefore your daily average). By mid-month, you should be totaling more than an hour a week, spread among your five days of jogging.

This means you will be *averaging* 12-15 minutes per day, which was your peak just a month before. Make this your main ambition—to turn last month's goal into this month's routine.

Also, try to push your longest jog up to 20-30 minutes or 2-3 miles—double your high of a month ago.

Jog at least 20 days this month, and walk informally on as many of the "rest" days as possible. This helps to strengthen the growing habit of daily exercise.

# Second Month's Jogging Plan

| Day | Suggested Training | Actual Training |
|---|---|---|
| 1 | 10-minute jog* | |
| 2 | rest** | |
| 3 | 5-minute jog | |
| 4 | 10-minute jog | |
| 5 | rest | |
| 6 | 5-minute jog | |
| 7 | 15-minute jog | |
| *Week's total of jogging (45 minutes):* | | |
| 8 | rest | |
| 9 | 10-minute jog | |
| 10 | 10-minute jog | |
| 11 | rest | |
| 12 | 10-minute jog | |
| 13 | 10-minute jog | |
| 14 | 20-minute jog | |
| *Week's total of jogging (60 minutes):* | | |

| Day | Suggested Training | Actual Training |
|---|---|---|
| 15 | rest | |
| 16 | 10-minute jog | |
| 17 | 15-minute jog | |
| 18 | rest | |
| 19 | 15-minute jog | |
| 20 | 10-minute jog | |
| 21 | 25-minute jog | |
| *Week's total of jogging (75 minutes):* | | |
| 22 | rest | |
| 23 | 10-minute jog | |
| 24 | 20-minute jog | |
| 25 | rest | |
| 26 | 20-minute jog | |
| 27 | 10-minute jog | |
| 28 | 30-minute jog | |
| *Week's total of jogging (90 minutes):* | | |

| Day | Suggested Training | Actual Training |
|---|---|---|
| 29 | makeup day*** | |
| 30 | makeup day | |
| 31 | makeup day | |

*Total number of training days for month (20):*______________

*Total amount of jogging for month (270 minutes):*____________

*Average jogging amount per day (13.5 minutes):*_____________

*Weight at beginning and end of month:*_____________________

*Resting pulse rate at beginning and end of month:*____________

(*all jogging this month is included in a total workout of 30 minutes or so, with the remainder of the time used for walking as warmup and recovery; **"rest" days should include some informal physical activity such as walking, bicycling, swimming; ***make up for sessions missed during the month)

# Lesson 14

# Forget the Myths

As you become a new runner, forget most of what you think you knew before about running, because most of it either isn't true or doesn't apply to the kind of running you're doing now.

If you're like most of the people who've grown up and left running behind, you still carry a mish-mash of impressions from a time when we all were runners.

Many of the leftover memories are negative. You remember when your mother shouted, "Don't run in the house!" You remember gym classes in which you ran lap after lap with no preparation and for no apparent purpose. You remember the high school football coach applying running as a punishment for minor breaches of discipline. You remember wearing 30 pounds of gear in the military and hearing the lightly-dressed drill sergeant command, "Double time, march!"

Or, if you once ran competitively, you think back on the drudgery of workouts—the monotonous routine of interval quarter-miles broken only by the anxiety, searing pain and exhaustion of the race.

For every good reason to start running, there are a half-dozen old memories saying why you shouldn't. The "why-nots" surround and devour a "why" each time it enters your head. This helps account for the fact that good intentions seldom translate into action.

Through the years you haven't been running, you've never considered that it might be anything but the way you remember

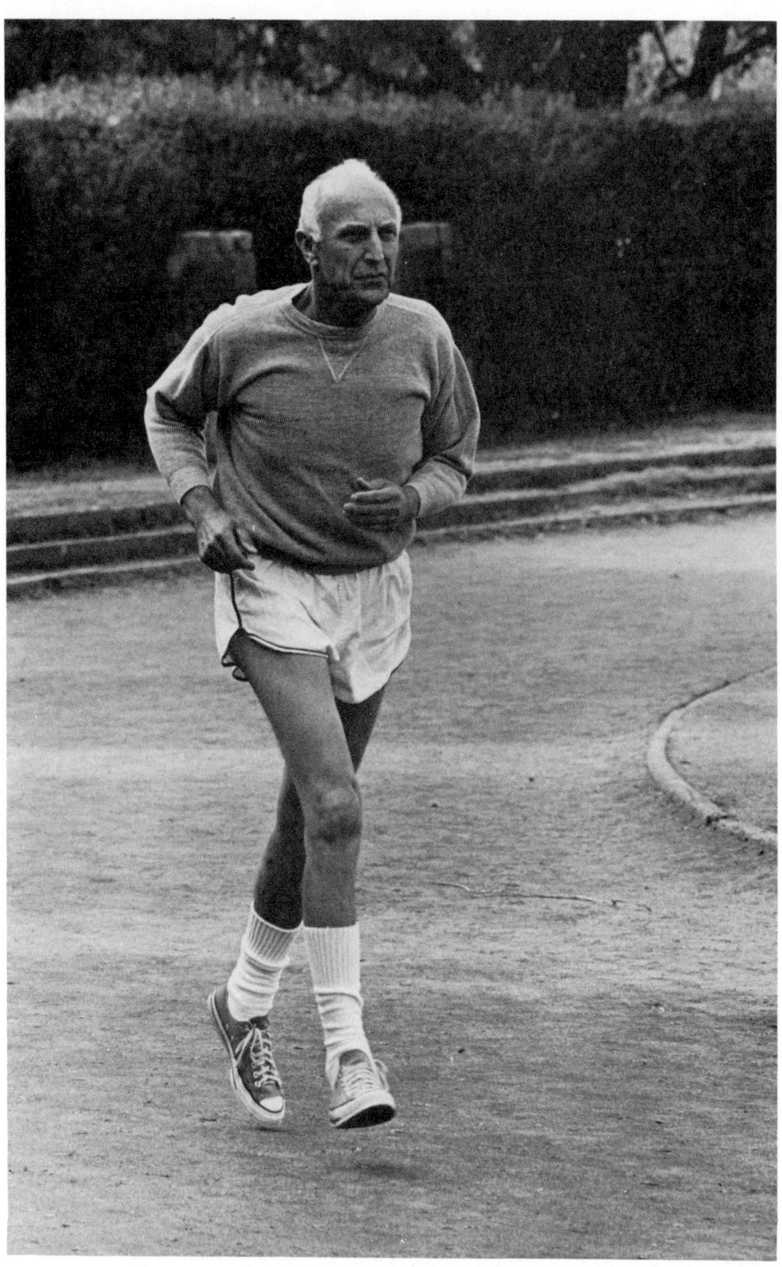

*"Nature returns to us in the persistence and staying power of maturity what she has taken away with the explosiveness of youth . . . ."*

it. You've never seen how darkly a few bad experiences have colored your impressions. You've never questioned the half-truths and myths about running which are spoken by people who don't run any more.

Before you can start running again and hope to keep running, you must clear away the debris left from any earlier experiences. Make a fresh start with a fresh set of ideas. Forget the old, negative ones. Forget the old associations of running with pain, punishment and pointlessness. Ignore the people who tell you what you can't do. Prove to yourself that the old limits don't hold you back any more.

Here are answers to the old assumptions about running which keep people from becoming runners. Perhaps some of them have held you back.

- **I don't have time.**

You don't need much. Ten to 20 minutes a day will put you in good enough shape for anything short of racing. If you're simply interested in a physical tuneup, you can't get a quicker one any other way.

An hour a week, divided among 3-6 days. That's all the time you need to invest. Most of us waste that hour and a lot more each day on extra sleep we don't need and on TV programs which wouldn't be missed.

Try filling the wasted minutes with running. Get up a little earlier in the morning. Turn on the TV a little later in the evening. Substitute a run for lunch. Don't wait for running time to open up. Make time.

- **I don't have a place to run.**

You don't need a special place. A school track is a luxury. If you live within a few blocks of one and you only plan to run a few laps, it's nice. But it isn't worth driving to if you're farther away, and its scenery gets old in a hurry.

A running place is anyplace. Wherever you can walk, you can run: parks, parking lots, bike paths, beaches, sidewalks, streets, schoolyards. Use whatever is available in your neighborhood. Choose quiet, pleasant-to-look-at routes over a variety of terrains and surfaces if you have a choice.

**• I don't have anyone to run with.**

This isn't tennis or softball. You don't need a partner or a team. You can go ahead alone, despite what your team-sport upbringing says otherwise.

In fact, once you break the old habit of leaning on others as you exercise and play, you probably will learn to like your independence. You can go where you want, when you want, at the pace you like. No more waiting for late partners. No more cancellations because teammates don't show up.

You learn to like setting your own schedule and talking to yourself as you carry it out. You become your own best companion.

**• I'm too old.**

Nonsense. If you think this, you've been brainwashed by the youth cult which has tried to tell us everything is downhill after 20.

The truth is, a runner's life has barely begun on his 20th birthday. The fastest of the distance runners are generally in their late 20s and early 30s. And there is evidence to show that endurance continues to grow in older runners even as speed is waning.

In other words, nature returns to us in the persistence and staying power of maturity what she has taken away with the explosiveness of youth. Kids are natural sprinters. The rest of us are natural endurance athletes.

**• I'm too weak.**

If you start telling me your physical limitations, I'll answer by telling you about the blind men who race marathons, or the runner who races on one leg, or the one who was born without feet. Or I'll tell you about the spreading use of running to rehabilitate heart attack victims.

One by one, the excuses for not getting active because of physical troubles are being shot down. So don't let yourself become a voluntary invalid because of minor complaints. Follow the example of runners who run through their serious problems. Practice active therapy.

**• It's too cold/too hot/too humid/too wet/too windy (pick one) to run.**

Regardless of appearances to the contrary, the human being wasn't born to live out his life in climate-controlled, air-conditioned, central-heated comfort. He's made with abilities to adapt to extremes of weather like those in Minnesota, where the winter-summer temperature variation is 100 degrees, yet runners never stop.

Running outdoors, year-round, is a chance to relearn those abilities. It's a chance to learn again to adapt with the changing seasons and to appreciate the subtle day-to-day changes you don't notice from indoors.

There will be bad days—perhaps more bad ones than good. But pushing through the bad ones will let you enjoy the good when they come. If you wait for perfect weather, you won't run very often.

**• It's boring.**

Running is boring only if you consider your own thoughts and the scene around you to be boring—only if you've been so thoroughly programmed by packaged thoughts and sights that you've forgotten how to do your own thinking and looking.

Experienced runners seldom talk of boredom. Instead, they talk of freeing themselves of cluttering thoughts, of doing their best creative work on the run, of seeing things on their routes which had never been apparent while driving there.

Boredom is related to fatigue and to impatience. Run within your limits, allow more than enough time for running, think and look while on the run, and you shouldn't be bored.

**• It's embarrassing.**

You're on your first run, and you feel the eyes of the world are on you. You wonder, what will the neighbors think? Why didn't I run at night so no one would see me? You've seen runners on these streets before, but you don't feel like one of them. You are too heavy, too clumsy. You aren't dressed right and aren't wearing the right shoes. You feel like an imposter.

At first, you try to hide your running as if it's something to be ashamed of. You leave the neighborhood for a hidden track, leave the daylight for the darkness, hide your legs under long pants, your arms under a jacket, your face under a hat.

But if you keep running long enough, you gradually realize the world's attention isn't centered on you. You develop pride in your running and don't care what anyone thinks. In fact, you wish more people would notice. You come out of the closet–back to the streets, back into the light of day, off with the camouflage.

- **It's dangerous.**

Everyone who runs or is thinking of running has heard of the dangers. He has seen the headlines: "Man, 46, Dies of Heart Attack while Jogging"; "Young Runner Struck by Auto, Seriously Injured"; "Competitors in Race Hospitalized for Heat Exhaustion."

Everyone hears the bad stories about running. The exceptions to the rules reach the papers. But no one reads of the thousands of people who have strengthened their ailing hearts and avoided attacks by running. No one reads of the thousands who run safely on the streets and in the heat.

Running isn't perfectly safe. But the precautions against trouble are so simple to take and the risks are so small that running should be considered no more dangerous than mowing the yard.

- **It's exhausting.**

If it is, you aren't doing it right. Only a competitive runner should ever exhaust himself, and he should be fit enough that he recovers quickly.

Your running routine is working if you can answer yes to these three questions:

1. Can I talk normally while I'm running?
2. Do I feel pleasantly tired, not wiped out, after I finish?
3. Am I free of soreness and carryover fatigue the next day, and eager to go again?

Find your own line between enough and too much running, and stay just a little on the low side of it. That's a basic rule in all training. "The harder you work, the better you'll be," and "It has to hurt to do any good," are myths.

# Lesson 15

# Speed Up

Dr. Kenneth Cooper has done more to get America moving than any politician could.

Back in the 1960s, Cooper was an Air Force medical officer. He'd tested his exercise ideas on thousands of airmen, and had written of the results in *Readers' Digest* and various Sunday supplements. Readers said, "Tell us more!" so he wrote the book *Aerobics.*

No fitness book has had a wider impact. This book and the two others which followed (*New Aerobics* and *Aerobics for Women*) have sold millions of copies. Millions of readers have taken their message to heart.

That message is: prolonged, steady-paced exercise is the surest path to cardiovascular fitness. And of the exercises, jogging and running give the quickest results.

In this lesson, I'm borrowing a few pages from Dr. Cooper because I can't construct any better jogging program than he already has. He tells his readers to jog at least four days each week. So do I. He tells them to average 1½-2 miles each of those days. I say about the same. He advises adding a little faster running. Now I'm going to let you do that, too.

You don't need to go any farther than you were going last month. In fact, if you're interested purely in reaching a satisfactory level of physical fitness in a short time, you *never* need to go any farther.

Dr. Cooper has a point system. I won't confuse you and myself with the scientific details, except to say that the system is scientifically based. It is his shorthand method for determining how much oxygen we use during exercise.

Cooper says we somehow need to accumulate 30 of these points each week to gain and maintain aerobic fitness. One mile at a moderate pace is worth about five points. Six miles a week equals 30 points. That totals only about an hour of jogging a week, and I already have you doing more than that.

The change this month is the addition of speed. You won't be racing, but I'm finally giving you the chance to run at a faster pace.

As always, you work into this gradually. You start by adding short "intervals" of running. Don't sprint. Don't make a sudden burst. Just slip from jogging into a faster rhythm. Stride smoothly and powerfully for no more than a minute, then slow to a walk for an equal amount of time before resuming jogging. The accelerations shouldn't exhaust you. The idea is to run them at a pace you will be able to hold for 12 minutes at the end of the month.

The 12-minute run is a standard Kenneth Cooper test. And by now you should be able to pass it with a "good" to "excellent" rating (see the accompanying chart). This is your goal for the month.

You may run either on a track or on a flat, carefully-measured road. The standard track is four laps to the mile. Five laps is 1.25 miles, six laps is 1.5 and seven laps is 1.75.

Warm up for the test with walking, jogging and short-distance running. Then have someone hold a watch for you, tell you when your 12 minutes are up and mark the distance completed.

Other goals for the month:

- Increase the amount of *running* each week (amount of jogging stays about the same).
- Train on at least 20 days.
- Jog-run an average of 15-20 minutes a day.
- Plan to continue with a similar or more advanced program after this one expires.

# Third Month's Jogging Plan

| Day | Suggested Training | Actual Training |
|---|---|---|
| 1 | 20-minute jog with one-minute run* | |
| 2 | rest** | |
| 3 | 10-minute jog | |
| 4 | 20-minute jog with one-minute run | |
| 5 | rest | |
| 6 | 10-minute jog | |
| 7 | 30-minute jog with one-minute run | |
| *Week's total of jogging-running (90 minutes):* | | |
| 8 | rest | |
| 9 | 10-minute jog with one-minute run | |
| 10 | 20-minute jog with 2x one-minute runs | |
| 11 | rest | |
| 12 | 20-minute jog with 2x one-minute runs | |
| 13 | 10-minute jog with one-minute run | |

| Day | Suggested Training | Actual Training |
|---|---|---|
| 14 | 30-minute jog with 2x one-minute runs | |
| *Week's total of jogging-running (90 minutes):* | | |
| 15 | rest | |
| 16 | 10-minute jog with one-minute run | |
| 17 | 20-minute jog with 3x one-minute runs | |
| 18 | rest | |
| 19 | 20-minute jog with 3x one-minute runs | |
| 20 | 10-minute jog with one-minute run | |
| 21 | 30-minute jog with 3x one-minute runs | |
| *Week's total of jogging-running (90 minutes):* | | |
| 22 | rest | |
| 23 | 10-minute jog with one-minute runs | |
| 24 | 20-minute jog with 3x one-minute runs | |

| Day | Suggested Training | Actual Training |
|---|---|---|
| 25 | rest | |
| 26 | 20-minute jog with 3x one-minute runs | |
| 27 | 10-minute jog with one-minute run | |
| 28 | 12-minute test*** | |
| *Week's total of jogging-running (90 minutes):* | | |
| 29 | makeup day**** | |
| 30 | makeup day | |
| 31 | makeup day | |

*Total number of training days for month (20):*____________

*Total amount of jogging-running for month (360 minutes):* ____________

*Average jogging-running amount per day (18 minutes):*__________

*Weight at beginning and end of month:* ____________

*Resting pulse rate at beginning and end of month:* ____________

(*the one-minute runs are not meant to be race-like but are somewhat faster than jogging pace; half-hour sessions now may include jogging, running and some walking; **"rest" days should include some informal physical activity; ***run as far as possible within the 12-minute limit; ****make up for sessions missed during the month)

## The 12-Minute Test

**Men** (distance in miles covered in 12 minutes)

| Fitness Category | Age 29-less | Age 30-39 | Age 40-49 | Age 50-up |
|---|---|---|---|---|
| Good | 1.50-1.74 | 1.40-1.64 | 1.30-1.54 | 1.25-1.49 |
| Excellent | 1.75-up | 1.65-up | 1.55-up | 1.50-up |

**Women** (distance in miles covered in 12 minutes)

| Fitness Category | Age 29-less | Age 30-39 | Age 40-49 | Age 50-up |
|---|---|---|---|---|
| Good | 1.35-1.64 | 1.25-1.54 | 1.15-1.44 | 1.05-1.34 |
| Excellent | 1.65-up | 1.55-up | 1.45-up | 1.35-up |

Your sex (men use top chart, women bottom) ____________

Your age (find appropriate column) ____________

Distance covered in 12 minutes ____________

Fitness rating (excellent, good or less) ____________

# Lesson 16

# Questions

- **Where is the best place to run?**

Anyplace you can safely walk will do for running. But some places are better than others. If you have a choice, look for running areas which meet as many of these criteria as possible:

1. Convenient enough that you can start and finish the runs at home. Don't waste time and trouble driving to a training site.
2. Relatively free of auto and pedestrian traffic. This cuts down on risk, bad air and self-consciousness.
3. Controlled dog population. Nothing ruins a run faster than a few unleashed dogs yapping at your heels.
4. Protection from wind and sun. Large shade trees along any route are a plus.
5. Few hills to climb. Advanced runners may seek out the mountains, but people who are content just to complete their daily distance quotas are happier on flat terrain.
6. Soft and smooth surfaces underfoot. Dirt and grass obviously are easier on the legs than asphalt and concrete, but rough ground can do as much damage to ankles and knees as hard surfaces can.
7. Pleasant to look at and hear. Natural sights and sounds are preferable to man-made ones.

Choose a variety of routes for a variety of reasons and seasons. It's a good way to get to know your town, for one thing. Also, you soon grow tired of a single path. Then, too, many of the best routes—the ones on softer ground—become impassible in snowy or rainy weather, and you need alternates.

There are several ways to lay out courses. Each has its advantages and limitations:

*Point-to-point*—Starting here, finishing over there someplace. It's most pleasant to run because there's no repeating, no circling back. It gives a natural feeling of "getting somewhere." But the problem is getting back again.

*Out-and-back*—Running to a turnaround point and then retracing your steps. It's the easiest type of route to follow when you aren't quite sure where you are. But some runners don't like to repeat themselves.

*Laps*—Going around and around the same circuit. A good way to run if you like to keep track of your pace along the way; not so good if you get bored easily.

*Loop*—A big circuit which starts and finishes in the same place but never covers the same ground twice. It eats up a lot of territory and may be hard to follow, but it probably is the all-round best way to lay out running courses.

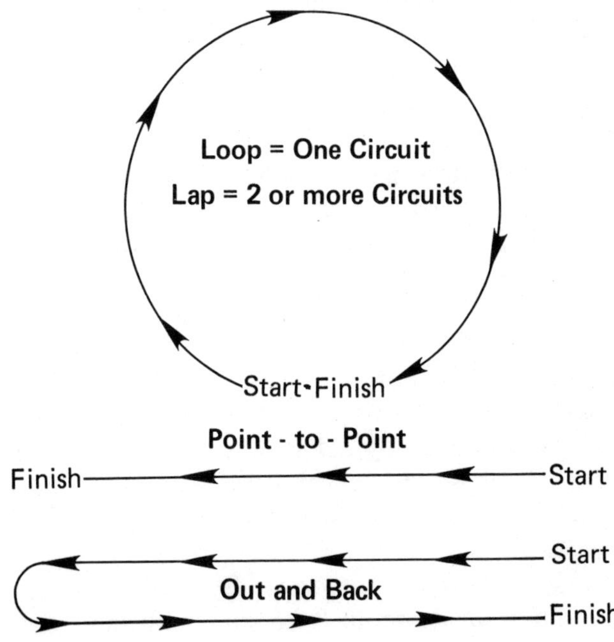

The easiest way to check a course's distance is with a car. Drive the route and measure it with the odometer (the distance counter). Be warned, though, that car measurements almost always produce short courses. Don't put much faith in the accuracy of times you run on these courses.

A better way to measure, if you want precision, is with a bicycle counter. This device fits on the front wheel of a bike. After it's calibrated over a measured course (such as a track), you can ride any route and find its distance within a yard per mile. (Alan Jones, 3717 Wildwood Dr., Endwell, N.Y. 13760 sells such a counter for about $12.)

- **When is the best time to run?**

Morning, noon or night, the effects are the same. When you run depends on the time of day when you operate best and when it's easiest for you to make time available for running.

You must *make* the time. We're all busy. We all can make the excuse, "I don't have time." No one can give you the time but yourself. Carve a chunk out of your day and make it sacred. Set aside a half-hour to an hour for yourself, and don't let anyone or anything intrude on it.

Some runners favor a first-thing-each-morning routine. Advantages: (1) seldom do other people and activities interfere at this time of day; (2) wakes you up for the day; (3) traffic is lightest; (4) air is cleanest and coolest. Disadvantages: (1) hard to roll out of bed, straight into a run; (2) you're sorest and stiffest at this hour; (3) it's dark and cold for a large part of the year.

Those who run in the evening or at night prefer it for these reasons: (1) they feel loosest and most wide awake then; (2) it calms them down after a day's hassles; (3) they like to run with other people, and it's easiest to find partners then. Minuses: (1) work and family obligations have a way of eating up this time; (2) winter nights get dark and cold early; (3) it's hard to delay supper when they come home hungry and still have a run to do.

One group of researchers who study such things found that morning runners are more likely to stick with the activity than those who run later. However, another group found that performance capacity is considerably better in the late afternoon and early evening. Take your pick.

Or run at noon. Noontime running is growing in popularity because it skips some of the negative aspects of morning and night: no darkness, no sleepiness or stiffness, few social obligations at this hour. Workers on a set schedule, with an hour off for lunch, find the time is better spent running than eating. The run blunts their appetite, gives them a physical break from mental fatigue and helps keep them awake all afternoon.

The problems with noontime running are: (1) finding a convenient place to run within close range of congested business or industrial areas; (2) finding a place to change for the run and shower afterwards.

These problems are being solved in areas where YMCAs, colleges, and parks and recreation departments are opening their facilities to runners at noon. Some progressive companies even are adding showers to encourage employee exercise.

A side-effect of this is "commute running." Workers who live within a convenient distance of the office or plant leave their cars at home and run to work, shower and dress there, then run home again at night. They get in two sessions of running and take only slightly more time than they would have needed to drive the distance.

However, this is an ambitious program recommended only for advanced runners with a high tolerance for a same-thing-every-day routine.

- **How do I set up a training plan?**

First, look back on what was said in answer to the last two questions—"where" and "when." Laying out routes and setting aside a time are the first two steps in programming your running.

You don't want to feel like a computer, mechanically responding to a pre-determined program. But a general, flexible plan for what you want to accomplish is important—particularly when you're new to running.

The plan is a raft to cling to when you otherwise might be lost in a sea of new and confusing information about this activity. It carries you through the risky places. It gives direction and continuity as you move toward a goal, and it is an intermediate goal in itself as you try to run as planned.

Plan to run with waves of effort. Not in a steady stream of same amount, same pace, same place every day, but by alternating harder runs and easier ones, long and short, work and recovery.

Schedule only three good, solid running days each week. Even if you run every day, emphasize just those three so you'll have time to recover from them. Put at least one easy or rest day between the harder ones. In other words, don't cram them together on Friday, Saturday and Sunday, then do nothing until the next Friday.

One possible arrangement is a Tuesday-Thursday-Saturday routine—with the best run of the week scheduled for Saturday when you generally have more time and energy. (Notice there are two days of recovery afterwards.)

Set a target number of miles for the week, or a total amount of time. Ten miles, 1½ hours; 50 miles, seven hours. The figure is up to you.

Now portion this amount out to the days of the week. If you're running just the minimum three days, your figuring is easy. Simply run about a third of the total each day. The rest days in between automatically take care of the hard-easy pattern.

If you prefer to keep running on most or all of the "easy" days, make the runs short. That might mean no more than half the distance or running time of the big days' sessions. This translates, for example, to four miles or so on the harder days and two miles or less on the easier ones.

Consider making one day each week—maybe Saturday—a really big one. Among runners, the weekend is a traditional time for extending distances or for testing speed.

You might want to try, on a weekend, to go up to twice as far as you usually go (for instance, eight miles if your typical distance is four) at a somewhat slower pace. Or you might want to time yourself at something below your normal distance.

Keep a log or diary to show where you have been and to give

you clues on where you are headed in your running. It's valuable as a record of how old plans were carried out, and as a guide on how new ones should be set up.

## Personal Schedule Planning

1. Decide on the total amount of time you plan to spend running each week or the total number of miles. __________

2. What is your number of training days weekly? __________

3. Figure the daily average needed to reach your quota (divide figure number one by figure two) __________

4. What is the projected length of the "short" runs (divide figure three in half) __________

5. How long should the "long" runs be? (Multiply figure three by two) __________

6. Approximate "collapse point" (average daily distance or time multiplied by three) __________

7. Weekly schedule:

   Day One (short run, see figure four*) __________

   Day Two (short run, see figure four*) __________

   Day Three (average run, see figure three) __________

   Day Four (short run, see figure four*) __________

   Day Five (average run, see figure three) __________

Day Six (short run, see figure four*) __________

Day Seven (long run, see figure five**) __________

*(*rest days may be substituted for one or more of the short days; **the "collapse point" shown in figure six should be considered as the upper limit of time or distance)*

8. Make increases in time at the rate of about 10% per run per week (add three minutes to a 30-minute run, six minutes to an hour run, etc.; list the amounts to be added to your short, average and long runs) __________ __________ __________

# PART FOUR

# RUNNING

# Lesson 17

# Introducing Running

You may never want to do any more than jog an average of 15 minutes or 1½-2 miles a day, four or five days a week. And there's no convincing physical reason why you should continue to advance.

You may remain a jogger and be proud of it. However, before you decide to level off in your efforts, listen to what I have to say about running. More precisely, about *fun*-running.

A few years ago, there really was only one way of looking at this activity. That was as a racer. About the only people who ran were the ones training for competition. They were serious because the only races were serious ones.

Then came the "Aerobics revolution" of the late 1960s and early '70s. Running had a new branch—jogging for fitness—and the number of people participating boomed.

But something was missing. The extremes—serious competition and simple fitness—were too far apart. Joggers found they got in shape rather quickly, and were looking for new challenges. Yet they didn't have the ability or inclination to compete seriously.

A middle level, fun-running, grew up to accommodate them. The fun-runner did more than the jogger but less than the top racer. The fun-runner competed, but his race was mostly against the distance and his own standards. Most importantly, he ran as much for his head as for his body from the neck down. He ran because he liked to run. He liked how it felt as he did it, and ran for that rather than as preparation for faraway rewards.

The differences among jogger, fun-runner and racer aren't measured so much in distance and speed as in attitude. There can be joggers who run six miles a day and fun-runners who go only three. Fun-runners can do 4:30 miles and sub-2:40 marathons, while racers struggle to reach slower times.

The differences are in the primary sources of their motivation—physical fitness, racing success or an attachment to running for its own sake.

I think everyone who runs can improve his outlook on the activity by learning from the fun-runner. If you only learn to like it a fraction as much as he does, you have gained. You have learned that running is worth holding onto. And this helps you get through the times when other goals seem too far away and too hard to reach.

The fun-runner's attachment, habit, addiction is the force which keeps pushing him out the door during those inevitable times when his will is weak. This season, nearly all the emphasis is on strengthening your attachment to running, solidifying your habit, forming an addiction.

Yes, I said "addiction." In fact, I used the word twice in the last paragraph so you wouldn't miss it. Runners do become addicted. Does that shock you? It shouldn't, because this addiction is a positive, perhaps even essential, type.

A number of reputable scientists have confirmed the presence and strength of this addiction. One doctor tested it several years ago, offering to pay runners not to run for a month. His first finding confirmed that something had a hold on them. Everyday runners refused to give up their exercise for any amount of money.

So the doctor settled for people who exercised just three times a week. Even they showed symptoms of lethargy, sleeplessness, tension and irritability when deprived of their usual activity.

These symptoms are common among runners who are forced to lay off for as little as a couple of days. Like an addiction to strong drugs, this running habit is both physical and psychological in origin. But unlike with drugs, there are no bad side-effects with running. Drugs weaken while exercise strengthens.

This is why Dr. William Glasser, a noted psychiatrist, calls

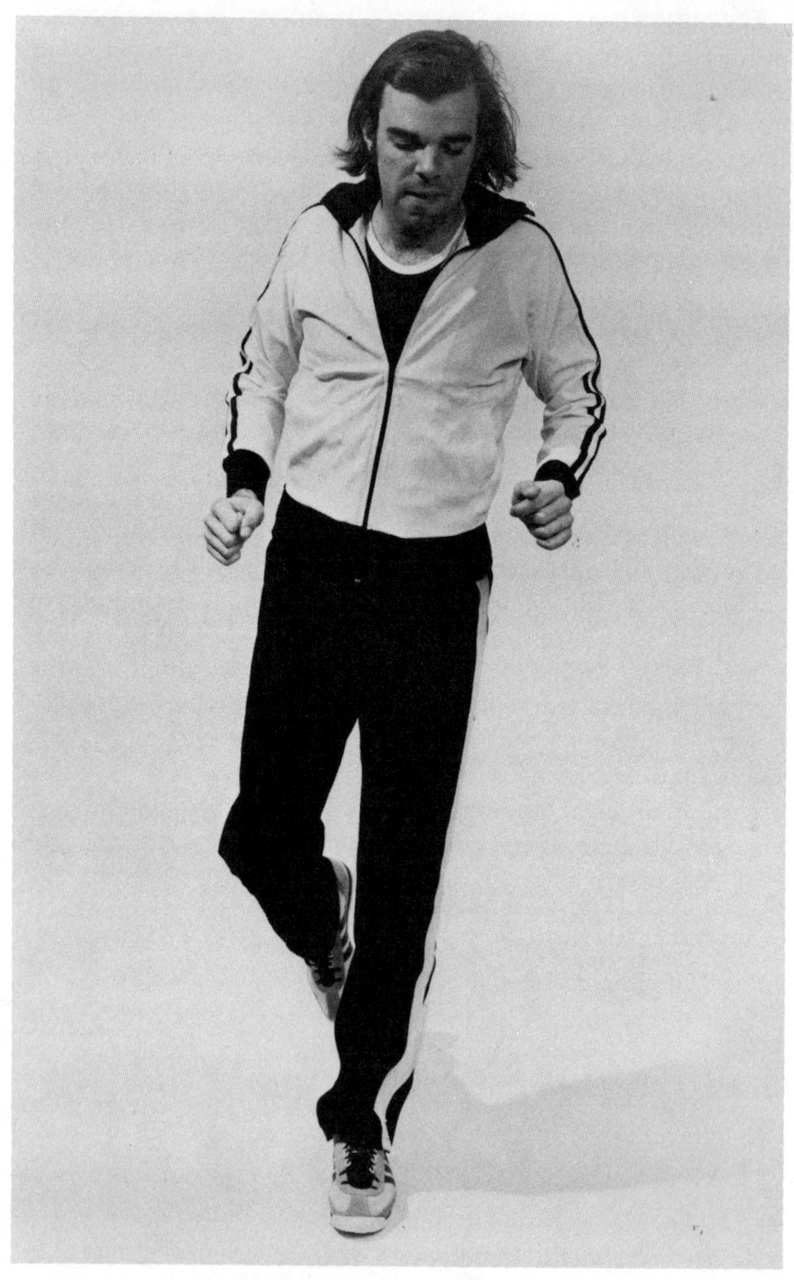

*"This season, nearly all the emphasis is on strengthening your attachment to running, solidifying your habit, forming an addiction . . . ."*

the running habit a "positive addiction." In a book by that title, he says running is the strongest of the positive addictions he has yet been able to identify, and he tells exactly how to achieve and recognize it.

In simplest terms, you form the habit by running long. It seems three miles or 20-30 minutes is the "addiction point" for most people. Once they're running that long each day, they're hooked. They know they're hooked when it bothers them more *not* to run than to get out and do it.

This season, I want you to concentrate on going longer. At least double the amount of running you were doing before. Discipline yourself to run three miles, 20-30 minutes or more nearly every day—until at the end of these months you don't have to think of it as "discipline" any more.

At the same time you are going longer, you are opening your eyes to all that running can be. Now that you aren't having to force each foot in front of the other, you have the chance to let your eyes and your mind wander as you run alone. You fall into step with other runners and find you have a lot of common ground to talk from. You find as you grow fitter you want to test the outer limits of your endurance and speed.

This season, for the first time, you get to sample the full diet of running:

- *Solo runs* in which you look at who and where you are.
- *Social runs* in which you talk with other runners who have had your experiences.
- *Speed runs* in which you race against your own limitations.

Like any diet, this one has to be properly balanced if it is to do the good it can.

The prerequisites for advancing from jogging to running are that you pass tests of general and specific fitness.

First, retake the fitness test in Lesson Four. By now, you will have wiped away most of your zero and one scores, and will have moved to several threes. Your total score probably is in the 20s, which it should be as you go running.

The second test, the Cooper 12-minute run, measures your

ability to combine endurance with speed. You are ready to run more and faster if you scored "good" to "excellent" in Lesson 15. Did you run 1½ miles or more (or the adjusted distance if you are over 30 years old or female) within the time limit? That should be thought of as the qualifying standard for running.

If you had trouble with either of the tests, repeat the third month of the jogging program (Lesson 15). Then test yourself again.

The running season follows the pattern which repeats itself throughout the book:

- *First month break-in.* Get used to running longer, and more often. Fix the running habit by eliminating most (if not all) days off, by cutting out most of the walking that remains and by running beyond the "addiction point" of three miles or 20-30 minutes every running day. Run gently and run alone, because the addiction forms quickest with slow, solitary running.

- *Second month build-up.* Extend your horizons. Once each week, go farther than you've ever gone before. Gradually push that distance out to 6-8 miles or one hour of running. Try to find someone to run with this day, and talk the miles away. If you can talk, you know you aren't working too hard. And as you run and talk, you draw strength from each other which totals more than the sum of its parts.

- *Third month speed-up.* Complete the running diet by working toward racing. Don't let the word "race" frighten you, because it won't be a national championship event, and you aren't required to beat anyone. You run with other people in distance races, but you compete only against yourself. That's the prevailing attitude in the sport. Having other people to lean on simply makes your race with yourself easier to bear and more meaningful. Work up to a three-mile or shorter race in the last week by adding brief "intervals" at racing pace each day, all month.

By the end of this season, you will have tasted nearly everything the running menu offers. And I hope you will have developed an appetite for it.

# Lesson 18

# Run Alone

The Big Lie on the physical side of running is, "If it is going to help you, it has to hurt." It is spread by people who confuse pain with purpose. The fact is, pain in running serves no purpose except to prevent you from inflicting more pain on yourself. It draws boundaries which you cross only at great risk.

I hope you've learned by now to run with a minimum of pain. And that you are becoming aware without my telling you that there is a Big Lie on the psychological side as well.

The second lie: "Running is, by its nature, a lonely and boring activity." This fallacy lives in the minds of people who confuse aloneness with loneliness and unstructured activity with boredom. They aren't the same. In fact, in many ways they are direct opposites.

The idea that the runner is lonely may trace to Alan Sillitoe, a British novelist. He wrote *The Loneliness of the Long-Distance Runner.* However, don't judge the book by its title. Sillitoe's hero wasn't lonely when he ran alone. He ran because of the loneliness he felt in the crowded city slums and in prison. He ran away from the crowd to look for himself. And he stopped running only when the crowd caught up with him and tried to make his running success their own.

Most of us who've run for a long time can identify with this character. I know I never feel more lonely than when I'm lost in a crowd; never more "together" than when I'm in the second half-hour of a run by myself. I'm never more bored than when I'm forced into an uncomfortable social role; never more inspired than when I'm free to let my feet and my thoughts ramble through a run.

A runner is a loner by necessity most of the time. I want to teach you here to be one by choice. Learn to like being alone. Cultivate aloneness as one of the hidden rewards of running instead of constantly seeking out partners as if this were a tennis match.

Get away from people and the talk they generate. All day long there is talk—talking out loud and talk on paper, live talk and canned talk.

You wake up in the morning to the news talk on the clock radio. You eat breakfast to the talk of the newspaper or the back of the cereal box.

All the day's work is a series of talking in conferences, sales negotiations, business luncheons, letters and reports.

You drive home each evening to the talk of the DJs on the car radio or the singers on the tape deck or the truckers on the CB. You talk to your family over dinner, and the TV talks to you until bedtime.

There's only one kind of talk missing from the day. You haven't left any time to talk with yourself. You haven't left yourself a quiet, uninterrupted hour with yourself in which to give your own ideas a good going over.

There is no shortage of talk in this turned-on, tuned-in world. But as the world grows busier and noisier, we let shrink that essential time each day to be alone to fantasize, to reflect, to clear away cluttering thoughts, to plan.

The beauty of running alone is that you can't take the outside talk with you, even if you want to carry it along. You must run away from family and friends, from TV and radio, from newspapers and books, from employees and bosses.

You run to no one's beat but your own. No one else is making you run. No one else cares whether you do it or not. The responsibility for running is yours entirely, and the same can be said for the rewards in doing it. They are all yours, too.

Five recommendations for learning to like running by yourself:

*1. Run away for an hour a day.* Don't expect to be given an hour. Make it. Squeeze it out of the busy day by combining wasted moments from elsewhere in your schedule. During that hour, separate yourself from all that is crowded, noisy or distracting. Be selfish with it because it is yours alone, and tolerate no intrusions on your time. Use the full hour for staying away from chaos, even if the hour is only half-filled with running.

*2. Don't hurt yourself.* Pain and boredom are closely linked. Pain "draws out the miles and makes them wearisome," to borrow words from Shakespeare. Runs that hurt are the ones that seem longest, and the ones you aren't anxious to repeat.

So don't push yourself too hard. Don't compete with yourself in training, because no matter how the race turns out, you lose. Run at a gentle pace which leaves you no more than pleasantly tired at the end–satisfied-with-the-effort, exhilarated tired, and not relieved-to-be-finished, exhausted tired.

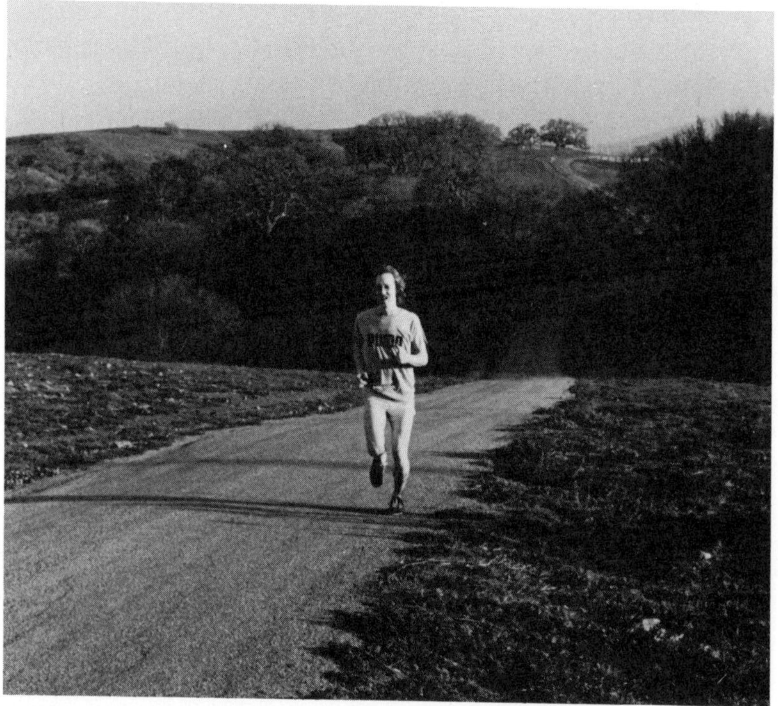

*"Learn to like being alone. Cultivate aloneness as one of the hidden rewards of running instead of constantly seeking out partners . . . ."*

*3. Wander.* Run free in both the physical and mental senses of the word. Have only the most general plan of where, how far and at what pace you want to go. Let your feet pick out the specifics according to how they feel as you go.

Have no preconceived notions about what your thoughts will be as you run. Intentionally avoid focussing on specific ideas. Let them float. Daydream.

*4. Meditate.* In the book I wrote before this one, I called running "moving meditation." If meditation describes types of thinking which lead to peace of mind, running fits the definition.

The steady, rhythmic beat of the feet replaces the chants used in more traditional meditation. There is the same sorting out of thoughts as they flow indiscriminately through your consciousness. (I described it in *The Long-Run Solution* as watching garbage go past on a conveyor belt. The good pieces are saved for recycling and the waste is carried away.) There is the same relaxed control of yourself afterwards.

*5. Create.* I don't literally write on the run. But I can say that if I didn't run, I wouldn't have much to say when I do write. I don't set out to think up story ideas and word combinations when I run. They just come. They come when I least expect them. They pop out of dark corners as I "daydream" and "meditate," and I use them later when I sit down to write.

The same will happen to you if you let it. A solution to a problem, a plan of action, an artistic inspiration will come to you once you clear your head.

Rarely can you do that when someone else is setting your running or conversational directions for you.

# Lesson 19

# Break In

The first 20 or 30 minutes of a run make a person fit. Most of the physical benefits can be had in that short time, and the returns diminish quickly from then on.

But it is the second 20 or 30 minutes that make running worth doing. That's when it starts to feel good and to make you glad you did the first part. The extra 20 or 30 minutes make you want to come back for more.

Dr. Thaddeus Kostrubala, a San Diego psychiatrist, uses running as psychotherapy with his patients. He has written a book titled *The Joy of Running*, and he says the joy is found late in a long run.

"The first 20 or 30 minutes, you feel rotten, fatigued, shot down," Kostrubala says. "Some in depression will actually cry. The draining feeling is emotional, not physical."

He says the depression disappears by 30 minutes and is replaced by "a distinct euphoria with feelings of excitement and enthusiasm." He calls it "the runner's high."

This may sound overstated if you haven't experienced the "high." But as one who feels it nearly every day, I can assure you that it is real and that it isn't really magic.

The first 20 minutes or so is simply a warmup. It takes that long to break out of your resting inertia, to break into a good sweat and to settle into a free-flowing rhythm and pace. It takes that long for your head to clear.

You obviously can get an adequate physical workout in less than 20 minutes, but you can't learn how a good run can feel in that little time. Because I believe a runner becomes positively addicted to that set of feelings, I recommend running well beyond 20 minutes until you don't want to do any less.

This month, work on the 20-30-minute habit. Work toward running almost as long every day as you ever went in previous months. The main goal of the month is to be averaging the 20-30 minutes a day by the last week.

Since you make something a habit by doing it every day, this month you should try to run daily. A few days off because of social conflicts, scheduling problems or minor aches and illness will be inevitable. But don't plan any layoffs. The sooner you work running in as a normal and comfortable part of your daily routine, the longer you'll stay with it.

Run alone on most of the days. Tune in to what you're feeling and thinking.

Be alert to any early signs of stress. They may appear since you're open to overstressing at times when the amount and frequency of running are climbing. Hold back on days when you have cold symptoms, hang-over fatigue from work the day before, heavy and stiff legs, and a general distaste for further exercise. If any leg pains increase as you go along in a run, stop. (Pains which go away as you warm up aren't usually so serious.)

Run at a gentle pace which allows you to complete your scheduled time or distance without struggling. See that your breathing stays normal, and keep your pulse rate below 150 as you run.

# First Month's Running Plan

| Day | Suggested Training | Actual Training |
|---|---|---|
| 1 | 10-minute run* | |
| 2 | 10-minute run | |
| 3 | 20-minute run | |
| 4 | 10-minute run | |
| 5 | 20-minute run | |
| 6 | 10-minute run | |
| 7 | 30-minute run | |
| *Daily average for first week (15 minutes):* | | |
| 8 | 10-minute run | |
| 9 | 10-minute run | |
| 10 | 25-minute run | |
| 11 | 10-minute run | |
| 12 | 25-minute run | |
| 13 | 10-minute run | |
| 14 | 35-minute run | |
| *Daily average for second week (17 minutes):* | | |

| Day | Suggested Training | Actual Training |
|---|---|---|
| 15 | 10-minute run | |
| 16 | 15-minute run | |
| 17 | 25-minute run | |
| 18 | 15-minute run | |
| 19 | 25-minute run | |
| 20 | 10-minute run | |
| 21 | 40-minute run | |
| *Daily average for third week (20 minutes):* | | |
| 22 | 15-minute run | |
| 23 | 15-minute run | |
| 24 | 30-minute run | |
| 25 | 15-minute run | |
| 26 | 30-minute run | |
| 27 | 15-minute run | |
| 28 | 45-minute run | |
| *Daily average for fourth week (23 minutes):* | | |

| Day | Suggested Training | Actual Training |
|---|---|---|
| 29 | makeup day** | |
| 30 | makeup day | |
| 31 | makeup day | |

*Total number of running days for month (28):*____________

*Total amount of running for month (540 minutes):*__________

*Average amount of running per day (19 minutes):*__________

(*it is recommended that all sessions be at least a half-hour, with walking making up the difference in time; **make up for sessions missed during the month)

# Lesson 20

# Run Together

My idea of torture is to stand among strangers at a party with a drink in my hand and a look of terror on my face, wondering what to say next and how to get away quickest. I seldom go to parties and I belong to no clubs. I work alone and I usually play alone. In short, I'm an archetypical runner in personality.

I talked, two lessons back, about the joys of being alone. And now I'm going to seem to contradict that by saying the highlight of my running and social week is my group run on Saturday mornings.

The advice in Lessons 18 and 19 was, "Run by yourself and not too fast." In this lesson and the next one, I say, "Run with someone else or a group, and not too fast." Then farther along I tell you, "Run with a group and go as fast as you can."

Confused? You may be, because there doesn't appear to be any consistency to my advice. Yet, hard as it may be to see, there is a method to it.

There is a time for each type of running–a time to think, to talk and to race. Each has its own purposes and benefits, and each eventually becomes a regular part of your schedule. You balance the three of them in a way which best suits your psyche.

I rarely saw another runner during my first four years of running. I learned to run alone and came to prefer it that way. So I still like doing my normal weekday distances by myself.

As I've aged, my appetite for competition has waned. Once, I needed to prove myself against the watch and against other runners several times a week. Now I feel the urge to race only about once a month—and then only in the most informal racing settings.

I run long once a week. By "long," I mean up to double my average for the other days of the week. That long run is the most valuable of my training week, but this is almost beside the point. Though I knew years ago that running this long would be good for me, I seldom did it. It seemed too far to go alone. Once I got beyond my familiar mileage range, I began looking for reasons to stop.

Now I rarely miss a long Saturday run, and very rarely stop early. I don't run long just because it's good for me but because this is a way to be with other people who think like I do. We draw ideas and strength from each other as we shrink the distances to be run.

Just as runners start to run alone because they must, and continue because they learn to like themselves, they sometimes come together for practical reasons and keep coming back for social ones.

The practical reason is mutual support. They can do distances together which they wouldn't be so likely to do alone. There is always that practical benefit to a group run, just as there is physical improvement during a run by yourself.

But the deeper you plunge into fun-running, the less important the physical returns are to you. They have value, of course, but are something like the gas mileage of your car. They are the by-product of having an efficient engine which is kept in good tune, but they have little to do with how much you enjoy your travels.

Just as running alone opens up time you might otherwise never take for traveling with yourself, running with others gives you time for talking you might otherwise never do.

There's something in the very act of running which encourages conversation, just as it coaxes out thought. Perhaps the gentle bouncing of the strides over long periods jars loose ideas we otherwise might have held inside.

Maybe the fact that when we are stripped down to run and all dressed the same makes all runners equal. We're symbolically stripped of the roles we carry the rest of the day. We're free of the verbal posturing we have to do the rest of the day.

In the group I run with, there are men and women. The age range is from pre-teens to mid-50s. At various times, we have engineers, business executives, blue-collar laborers, housewives, students, doctors, lawyers, salesmen, teachers and editors in the group.

Rarely would people who seem this different get together at any other time. But rarely do their differences matter when we run. We don't talk of ages or sexes or occupations because they don't matter during this two hours on Saturday mornings. We talk mainly about running, because it is the one thing we all have in common.

The reason we like being together and why the talk flows so freely may simply be this: It's the one time each week when we can talk about a subject important to us with people who understand and care. We can say what we want about our running and be greeted by nods of agreement rather than by vacant stares or you-must-be-crazy shakes of the head.

Runners share a secret. We know we may look and act a little weird by the standards of the sitdown world, but we know too that our running is setting free the thoughts, words and sensations which stagnate in non-movers.

Because we share this secret, no runner is a stranger to any other. A runner from Boston and one from Auckland can meet on a street in Los Angeles and be talking like old friends inside of five minutes because they are talking from common groups.

If a person who's basically a loner like me can call his occasional group run "the social highlight of my week," anyone can. I've run with my group nearly every Saturday for five years. The group has stayed together that long because of the way it works. Other groups could work the same way. Here's how:

1. *Make it practical.* Offer something in the group run which a runner can't or won't do alone. Not the talk, though it is important. I mean have a practical *running* reason to come to-

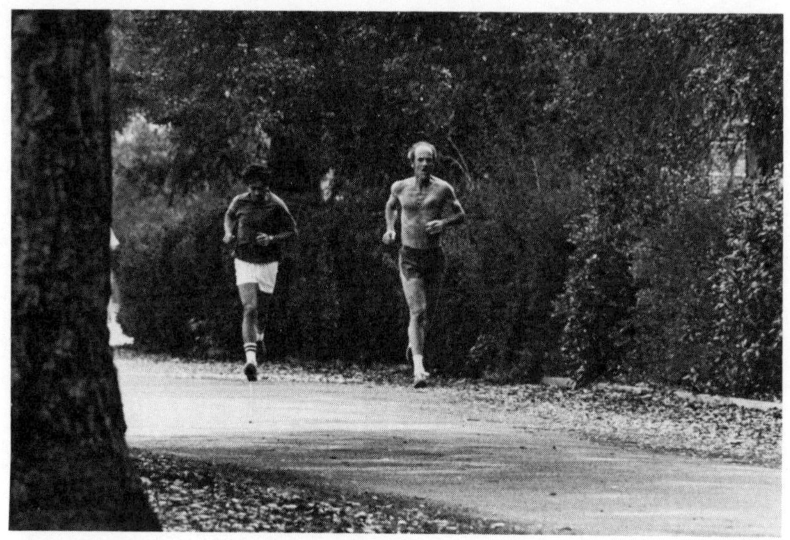

*"Just as running alone opens up time for traveling with yourself, running with others gives you time for talking you might otherwise never do. . . ."*

gether, like this being the longest and hardest run of the week. Having other runners along makes it seem shorter and easier.

2. *Keep it small.* A "group" may just be you and someone else. That's okay. That's the easiest kind of group to put together. Three or four people are better, because if one is gone the group still goes on. With five or more, it starts getting unwieldy and impersonal. You have a hard time agreeing on where and how fast to go, and what to talk about.

3. *Think and act alike.* Members of the group should be about the same in abilities and ambitions. Nothing splits a group quicker than disagreements over distances and paces.

4. *Be regular.* Have a common, agreed-upon meeting place and time. For instance, every Saturday morning, eight o'clock, in the school parking lot. This way, no one has to make any arrangements to see that everyone gets there.

5. *Set your routes.* Establish one or more standard running courses of the type and distance you prefer. Make sure they are safe, rather scenic, and are easily followed. And see that everyone in the group knows the way. Then no one will get lost if he strays from the pack.

6. *Stay together.* The only purpose of a group run is to help each other and talk with each other. If it quickly splits up and the runners are 100 yards apart, it serves no purpose. You might as well have started alone. Run at the pace of the slowest runner in the group—or if the slowest one falls off the group's pace, circle back to pick him up. The slowest runner is the one who needs the group's support the most.

7. *Talk.* Talking is, of course, one of the two reasons for being together. But it also a test. It's a way of letting you know that you're staying within speed limits. As long as you want to and can talk, you aren't running too hard.

8. *Don't race.* Racing the long distances destroys the group two ways. First, it splits it up into an every-man-for-himself struggle. And then it grinds each man down. You have gained little if you go twice as far on Saturday as you normally run but are so tired the next six days that you do only half of normal. Run gently when you run long. Save the speed for another day. Savor the people and the distance, don't fight them.

# Lesson 21

# Build Up

"Long," like "fast," is a relative term, based on what you're used to doing, and you may think you're going long enough already. But I want you to try to go longer precisely because this feeling of distance is so relative. By running longer, you make what used to be long seem shorter.

Years ago, when I began to go long, I thought the best way to do it was to run the same distance every day of the week. In my case, I wanted to do 50 miles a week, so I put in exactly seven a day and picked up the extra mile someplace.

This got to be a grind because there never was any variety, never any contrasts, never any hard or easy days. Because I had nothing to compare them to, all the runs seemed long.

I still do about 50 miles a week, but I almost never run seven miles. Some days it's a lot more than that, some a lot less. If I do run seven, it isn't at all imposing because I regularly go twice that far. I'm able to handle something as long as that because I know a couple of recovery days will follow.

The weekly long run is the glue which holds the rest of my week together. It consolidates everything I do the other six days and makes it all seem as easy as strolling around the block.

Learning to run longer is above all a matter of pacing. Run slowly enough to let yourself go long. (I had a racing background when I started extending my distances, and it was months before I could slow down enough to reach 10 miles.) Keep the breathing normal and the pulse below 150.

Move ahead by small steps. You can expect to handle comfortably about a 10% increase in time or distance each week. For example, if your longest is 40 minutes, 10% of that is four minutes. Step up to 44. If you're at a five-mile plateau, add a half-mile. Resist the temptation to go too far, too fast, too soon.

It's obvious that a runner has speed limits. You can only go so fast before nature stops you. But we also have distance limits which aren't so obvious. Most runners figure, "If I go slow enough, I can run forever." Not true.

Training sets a limit of how far you can run. This is called the "collapse point," the point at which all your reserves are drained and you have a hard time even getting your feet off the ground. Runners generally "collapse" at about three times their average daily time or distance. So if you average 30 minutes or four miles, your limits are 1½ hours or 12 miles.

Don't press that limit too closely. Keep the long run within 1½ to two times your average. Make it your first goal for the month to extend your longest run to an hour or more (it doesn't matter how much distance you cover in that time as long as you run for a full hour).

The second goal is to pull up your average to a half-hour or more per day by the end of the month. Count up all your running time and divide it by the number of running days at the end of each week. Try to increase the amount by a few minutes per week.

# Second Month's Running Plan

| Day | Suggested Training | Actual Training |
|---|---|---|
| 1 | 15-minute run* | |
| 2 | 15-minute run | |
| 3 | 35-minute run | |
| 4 | 15-minute run | |
| 5 | 35-minute run | |
| 6 | 15-minute run | |
| 7 | 45-minute run | |
| *Daily average for first week (25 minutes):* | | |
| 8 | 15-minute run | |
| 9 | 15-minute run | |
| 10 | 40-minute run | |
| 11 | 15-minute run | |
| 12 | 40-minute run | |
| 13 | 15-minute run | |
| 14 | 50-minute run | |
| *Daily average for second week (27 minutes):* | | |

| Day | Suggested Training | Actual Training |
|---|---|---|
| 15 | 20-minute run | |
| 16 | 20-minute run | |
| 17 | 40-minute run | |
| 18 | 20-minute run | |
| 19 | 40-minute run | |
| 20 | 20-minute run | |
| 21 | 50-minute run | |
| *Daily average for third week (30 minutes):* | | |
| 22 | 20-minute run | |
| 23 | 20-minute run | |
| 24 | 40-minute run | |
| 25 | 20-minute run | |
| 26 | 40-minute run | |
| 27 | 20-minute run | |
| 28 | One-hour run | |
| *Daily average for fourth week (31 minutes):* | | |

| Day | Suggested Training | Actual Training |
|---|---|---|
| 29 | makeup day** | |
| 30 | makeup day | |
| 31 | makeup day | |

*Total number of running days for month (28):*____________

*Total amount of running for month (795 minutes):*_________

*Average amount of running per day (28 minutes):*__________

(*it is recommended that all sessions be at least a half-hour, with walking making up the difference in time; **make up for sessions missed during the month)

# Lesson 22

# Run Fast

The separation between "jogging" and "running" is a rather artificial one, involving subtle differences in pace and attitude. I try not to make too much of these differences, because they tend to put people into arbitrary categories from which they have a hard time escaping.

If you're looking for a division in this sport, the real one is between "running" and "racing." They are as different as a Sunday drive is from the Grand Prix of Monaco.

Running works on physical and mental fitness. Racing works on the ego.

Running builds you up physically. Racing may tear you down.

You run best when you cooperate with yourself and your environment, coaxing out the benefits. You race best when you work against your natural instincts to slow down and avoid pain. In racing, you make a direct challenge to distance, time, terrain and other racers.

The pleasure in running is in the doing and in the immediate after-effects. The pleasure in racing is in the anticipation of racing, before the pre-race nerves set in, and in the reflection after you have recovered from the event.

Racing is a panicky dash which you can't wait to finish. It's painful before, during and after. It contributes little or nothing to fitness, and indeed may work against it by straining you to the breaking point.

Knowing this, you might be asking now, "Why bother? Why

should I subject myself to so much suffering for something I don't even need?"

No one needs to race. No one needs to suffer in running to get most of its benefits. If you don't feel like racing and suffering, don't bother. I admire you for your restraint.

That's something I've never had. Even though I'm basically a runner who paces myself comfortably, I regularly get the itch to push. Ninety-five per cent of my running is gently paced, but I have raced more than 500 times to satisfy that itch.

Most days, I'm content to ramble around the familiar plains of the sport. But sometimes I want to explore its peaks and valleys. This climbing up and falling down is hard and painful, but it is good for my ego in a way everyday running can never be.

Racing is where I have to face the truth about myself. In a gentle run, I can fool myself. When I'm cruising at well below maximum effort, my pictures of my capabilities are easily distorted.

But racing doesn't lie. It tells me exactly what I can do. Occasionally, I can do what I thought I could. But usually it is something more or less. Whether the race teaches me pride or humility, it tells me the truth.

Running is having fun. It is an escape into euphoria. Racing is facing the reality of pain and possible failure while chasing dreams.

Racing is a voluntary act of self-abuse. Before you decide to do it, you must be very sure this is what you want. Once you're sure of that, approach your first race warily. Plot your path of approach carefully and tiptoe along it, or you will crush yourself while trying to become a more complete runner.

Some hints for smoothing the path to your first race:

1. *Preparation.* This runs in two directions. First, you need the endurance to cover the distance comfortably. Experienced marathoners say the minimum is a third of the race distance per day as an average. But you aren't starting with a marathon. You should be racing a far shorter distance and be averaging at least that *full* distance per day. Then you know you can go far enough.

Second, you learn to go fast enough. Practice running small portions of the racing distance at the top pace of the race. Then in the race you can combine distance and speed.

2. *Competition.* Beginning racers have an exaggerated fear of competition. They think everyone will run away from them, that they'll finish last and that everyone else will laugh. Don't believe it. Distance racing isn't like that.

For one thing, it is open to everyone. Most races have people who run all the way from sub-five-minute to 10-minute-plus miles. It's almost impossible to be by yourself even if you want to be, and it's hard to be last even if you try.

In all my years of going to road races, I've never known anyone to finish last. Of course, someone has to take the final spot, but he's often as happy as the first placer, so no one can call him a loser.

Don't worry about anyone laughing at you. Not only will you have lots of company in the middle or at the back of the pack, but you'll find the people around you are friendly and helpful. This is how it is in distance racing. The real competition isn't with each other but with yourself and the distance, and having company makes that race easier.

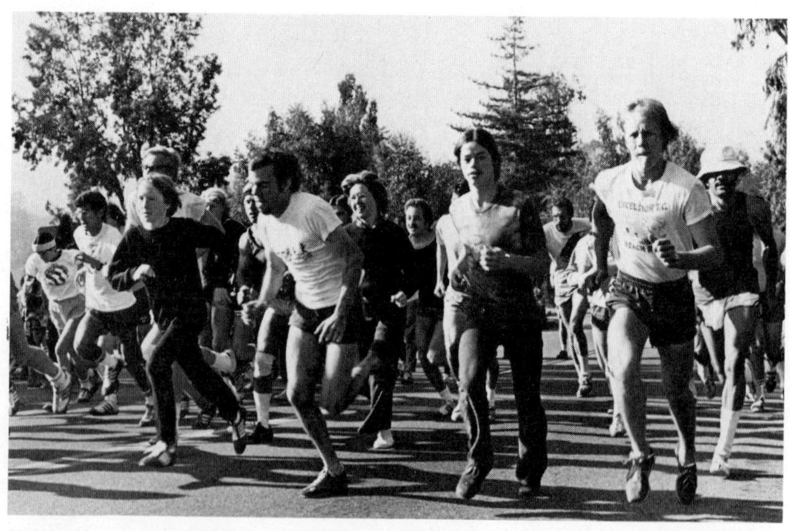

*"The best place to begin racing is at a Fun-Run. This is competition at the most informal level . . . ."*

3. *The Race.* The best place to begin racing is at a Fun-Run. This is competition at the most informal level, so it isn't as frightening as bigger events might be. No group membership is required. There are no entry fees, no registration of entrants and no prizes. A group of runners simply gets together to race a measured distance against time. If nothing like this is going on now in your area, you and your running friends can easily set up a Fun-Run of your own.

Keep the first race within your distance and speed ranges. If you've followed the schedules in this book, you are not ready to try either a race longer than 10 miles or an all-out dash of less than a mile. Your training best suits you for something in the 2-5-mile range.

4. *Pacing.* The temptation, when you get with a group of racers, is to explode away from the starting line—to go as fast as you can for as long as you can. Resist it. Work against your natural urges by holding back when you feel like letting go and later by pushing when you feel like slowing down.

Try to make the second half of the race faster than the first. That means you'll be passing people who spurted away from you at the start. You'll have the good feeling of finishing strongly instead of struggling home.

5. *Attitudes.* I've already talked about the most important one. That is, you're competing with yourself and can win no matter where you finish.

Two other attitudes will help: Realize it's normal to feel anxious and uncertain as you approach a race, because your nerves are getting you ready for hard work which you couldn't handle if you were calm. And accept the temporary pain that goes with racing effort, because overcoming pain makes racing worthwhile.

# Lesson 23

## Speed Up

Start the new month with a second 12-minute test. Lesson 15 tells how it's done. Your improvement since the first one should be rather dramatic, since you've had at least two months of longer-distance training since the last test.

However, the improvement in those months won't be nearly as great as the progress you'll notice in the next few weeks. I don't want you to make this a goal, necessarily. But from the test at the first of the month to the race at the end, I expect you will increase the distance you can go at a particular pace. For instance, if you tested out at a mile and a half in 12 minutes, you probably will race three miles in 24 minutes.

There will be two reasons for the quick improvement: (1) the other people in the race will pull you along farther and faster than you could go alone, and (2) for the first time, you will be training to race.

Up to now, the emphasis has been on slow-paced endurance running, on building up your distances and on exercising caution. I don't want you to forget these lessons, since they still make up more than nine-tenths of your routine. But now you are free to add some speed.

Before you race, practice running at race pace. Play with speed before you have to work at it. Use "fartlek." This rather gross-sounding word is Swedish for "speed-play."

In its pure form, fartlek involves running across the fields and through the woods, adding variations of pace at will and never timing anything.

I prefer a more formal variation of fartlek, because most runners seem to need more direction and goals than this free-form training gives. My variation involves blending short bursts of speed at about racing pace into an otherwise long and gentle run. The accelerations may be on a track or other measured course but usually are done wherever you happen to be at the moment. They may be timed but usually are run at a pace which "feels" right.

Make the fast running no more than one-tenth of the day's total. I personally favor one-twentieth, and use this formula in the accompanying schedules. This amounts to one minute in every 20. If you go an hour, add three fast minutes.

Divide the fast running up into several segments. For instance, do three bursts of a minute each, with plenty of recovery time in between. And don't time them. Just accelerate smoothly until you reach a pace which seems about fast enough for racing, then hold it for the allotted time. Don't try to run them any faster than you think you will be racing. This is *preparation* for racing, not racing itself.

Your goal for the month is simply to get ready for the race at the end and to complete it in a way which satisfies you.

## Third Month's Running Plan

| Day | Suggested Training | Actual Training |
|---|---|---|
| 1 | 20-minute run* | |
| 2 | 20-minute run | |
| 3 | 40-minute run with one minute at race pace** | |
| 4 | 20-minute run | |
| 5 | 40-minute run with one minute at race pace | |
| 6 | 20-minute run | |
| 7 | 12-minute test*** | |
| *Daily average for first week (27 minutes):* | | |
| 8 | 20-minute run with one minute at race pace | |
| 9 | 20-minute run with one minute at race pace | |
| 10 | 40-minute run with 2 x one minute at race pace | |

| Day | Suggested Training | Actual Training |
|---|---|---|
| 11 | 20-minute run with one minute at race pace | |
| 12 | 40-minute run with 2 x one minute at race pace | |
| 13 | 20-minute run with one minute at race pace | |
| 14 | One-hour run with 3 x one minute at race pace | |
| *Daily average for second week (31 minutes):* | | |
| 15 | 20-minute run with one minute at race pace | |
| 16 | 20-minute run with one minute at race pace | |
| 17 | 40-minute run with 2 x one minute at race pace | |
| 18 | 20-minute run with one minute at race pace | |

| Day | Suggested Training | Actual Training |
|---|---|---|
| 19 | 40-minute run with 2 x one minute at race pace | |
| 20 | 20-minute run with one minute at race pace | |
| 21 | One-hour run with 3 x one minute at race pace | |
| *Daily average for third week (31 minutes):* | | |
| 22 | 20-minute run with one minute at race pace | |
| 23 | 20-minute run with one minute at race pace | |
| 24 | 40-minute run with 2 x one minute at race pace | |
| 25 | 20-minute run with one minute at race pace | |
| 26 | 40-minute run with 2 x one minute at race pace | |

| Day | Suggested Training | Actual Training |
| --- | --- | --- |
| 27 | 20-minute run with one minute at race pace | |
| 28 | 3-mile race or time trial | |
| *Daily average for fourth week (27 minutes):* | | |
| 29 | makeup day*** | |
| 30 | makeup day | |
| 31 | makeup day | |

*Total number of running days for month (28):*__________

*Total amount of running for month (820 minutes):*__________

*Average amount of running per day (29 minutes):*__________

(*it is recommended that all sessions be at least a half-hour, with walking making up the difference in time; **run at about the pace you expect to go in the race at the end of the month; ***make up for sessions missed during the month)

# Lesson 24

# Questions

- **What type of diet should a runner follow?**

The sport has the reputation, with good reason, of being a haven for diet faddists of every persuasion. Runners have the feeling that somewhere, sometime they'll find the super diet which suddenly will transform them into super runners. They think their running dreams are as close as the end of a fork.

They could be right, but I doubt it. I haven't seen many hints in the last 20 years that this is true, but I'm not posing as an expert on nutrition. If you're seriously interested in shaping up your diet, buy a general nutrition book. It doesn't matter if the book isn't written for runners, because runners' dietary needs probably aren't much different than anyone else's.

Only make changes in eating and drinking habits if they contribute to overall health. Don't fall into the trap of thinking you'll be a better runner simply by eating better. At best, eating right only gives you a foundation of good health on which to put more training.

But you still have to do the training. As a runner, you are what you *run*, not what you eat. Dietary practice may smooth or block the path of running, but they don't provide any shortcuts.

Runners gulp down honey and avoid white sugar as if it were rat poison. Some take protein supplements while others restrict their protein intake. Some eat only natural, unprocessed foods while others eat from pill bottles. Sometimes they eat six small meals a day, sometimes only a single big one.

# Caloric Cost of Running

| CALORIES USED PER MILE OF RUNNING | | | | | | | | | |
|---|---|---|---|---|---|---|---|---|---|
| WEIGHT | PACE PER MILE | | | | | | | | |
| (pounds) | 5:20 | 6:00 | 6:40 | 7:20 | 8:00 | 8:40 | 9:20 | 10:00 | 10:40 |
| 120 | 83 | 83 | 81 | 80 | 79 | 78 | 77 | 76 | 75 |
| 130 | 90 | 89 | 88 | 87 | 85 | 84 | 83 | 82 | 81 |
| 140 | 97 | 95 | 94 | 93 | 92 | 91 | 89 | 88 | 87 |
| 150 | 103 | 102 | 101 | 99 | 98 | 97 | 95 | 94 | 93 |
| 160 | 110 | 109 | 107 | 106 | 104 | 103 | 101 | 100 | 99 |
| 170 | 117 | 115 | 113 | 112 | 111 | 109 | 107 | 106 | 105 |
| 180 | 123 | 121 | 120 | 119 | 117 | 115 | 114 | 112 | 111 |
| 190 | 130 | 128 | 127 | 125 | 123 | 121 | 120 | 118 | 117 |
| 200 | 137 | 135 | 133 | 131 | 129 | 128 | 126 | 124 | 123 |
| 210 | 143 | 141 | 139 | 137 | 136 | 134 | 132 | 130 | 129 |
| 220 | 150 | 148 | 146 | 144 | 142 | 140 | 138 | 136 | 135 |

**Note:** expenditure of 3500 calories equals one-pound weight loss.

| CALORIES USED PER MINUTE | | | | | | | | | |
|---|---|---|---|---|---|---|---|---|---|
| WEIGHT | PACE PER MILE | | | | | | | | |
| (pounds) | 5:20 | 6:00 | 6:40 | 7:20 | 8:00 | 8:40 | 9:20 | 10:00 | 10:40 |
| 120 | 15.6 | 13.8 | 12.1 | 10.9 | 9.9 | 9.0 | 8.3 | 7.6 | 7.0 |
| 130 | 16.9 | 14.8 | 13.2 | 11.8 | 10.7 | 9.7 | 8.9 | 8.2 | 7.6 |
| 140 | 18.1 | 15.9 | 14.1 | 12.6 | 11.5 | 10.5 | 9.6 | 8.8 | 8.1 |
| 150 | 19.4 | 17.0 | 15.1 | 13.5 | 12.3 | 11.2 | 10.2 | 9.4 | 8.7 |
| 160 | 20.6 | 18.1 | 16.1 | 14.5 | 13.0 | 11.8 | 10.9 | 10.0 | 9.3 |
| 170 | 21.9 | 19.2 | 17.0 | 15.3 | 13.8 | 12.7 | 11.5 | 10.6 | 9.8 |
| 180 | 23.1 | 20.2 | 18.0 | 16.2 | 14.6 | 13.3 | 12.2 | 11.2 | 10.4 |
| 190 | 24.4 | 21.3 | 19.0 | 17.0 | 15.4 | 14.0 | 12.9 | 11.8 | 10.9 |
| 200 | 25.6 | 22.4 | 19.9 | 17.9 | 16.2 | 14.8 | 13.5 | 12.4 | 11.5 |
| 210 | 26.9 | 23.6 | 20.9 | 18.7 | 17.0 | 15.5 | 14.1 | 13.0 | 12.1 |
| 220 | 28.1 | 24.7 | 21.9 | 19.6 | 17.8 | 16.2 | 14.8 | 13.6 | 12.6 |

I've been to all of these extremes and back, and as far as I can tell none of them makes any measurable difference in running performance. The differences don't seem to come from what I eat but from how much and when.

Without question, quantity has the most direct influence on running. How much you eat determines how much you weigh, and your weight is what you carry with you. The less excess baggage you carry, the easier you run.

After you've been running a while, you don't need a scale to tell you you're a few pounds overweight. You feel the extra burden as surely as if you were wearing a weighted belt.

Keep track of your weight. Weigh yourself daily and weekly under constant conditions, and trim away little gains before they grow into big ones.

You occasionally will dip well under your ideal weight, too. This usually happens in hot weather. Assume with all sudden drops in weight that you're running a water deficit. You've sweat away too much and haven't replaced it. If you're down a few pounds in weight, give it a chance to come back to normal before running long or hard again.

When to eat? Look at it this way. Anything you're carrying in your stomach, no matter how nutritious, isn't going to help any on this run. But it can hurt. It can lead to stomach cramps, side "stitches," unscheduled pit stops or even vomiting.

I've never collapsed from malnutrition during a run (though I regularly run 6-12 hours after my last meal), and I've never seen it happen to anyone else. However, I've experienced all the effects of eating too close to a run. So it seems wiser to run empty. You aren't a car, and your fuel isn't stored in a tank. It's out in the muscles as the result of food eaten much earlier.

- **What do I do if I'm injured or ill?**

Conventional medical wisdom is, "Stop running until you get well." But this advice doesn't take into account the runner's "addiction" and the fact that a week off makes him more miserable than the ailment.

Therefore, the best medical care for a runner is *prevention.* Run in a way which minimizes the chances of getting hurt or ill. Be alert to problems in any of four areas:

1. *Overwork*–more stress than you can handle at the moment.

2. *Faulty equipment*–shoes which are inadequate for your purposes or are too badly worn to protect you.

3. *Muscle tightness*—running is a "tightening" activity, and most runners need to loosen up with supplementary exercises.

4. *Form faults*–stress caused by the way your feet hit the ground.

Form faults can be taken care of partly through attention to running techniques (see Lesson Eight). But if they're related to structural quirks–flat feet, for instance–you may need help from a doctor who makes corrective supports.

Muscle-loosening exercises are described in answer to the next question of this lesson. Ideally, you should balance off each running workout with a set of these exercises.

Lesson Eight talks about the kind of shoes a runner needs. Give special attention to the heel construction and forefoot flexibility of the shoes you buy, because defects here are major injury producers.

Of all the sources of trouble, however, overwork is the key one. You may get by on bad feet, bad shoes and tight muscles if your workload is right. But a little bit too much stress will find your breaking point, whether it be injury or illness.

Everyone has these breaking points. We uncover our weaknesses when we suddenly plunge into new and harder types of running, or when we forget that rest and recovery are as much a part of the training formula as hard work is.

The human body cooperates in preventive medicine. It gives early warning signs when something is going wrong, and we must pay attention. Chronic, low-grade leg soreness and stiffness, cold symptoms, lingering fatigue, listlessness and psychological unrest are gentle reminders to back off. You're no longer training; you're straining. And the warnings will get progressively less gentle if you refuse to heed them now.

Serious running ailments need not happen. They do happen, of course, but they can be prevented if you are flexible in every sense of the word. Flexibility of the muscles is important, yes, but flexibility of the *mind* is much more so. Bend your running schedule to fit your feelings, not the other way around.

If you spot the symptoms early, you rarely will need to stop running to get rid of them. Simply cutting back on amount and intensity of training for a few days will take care of most problems.

Only in extreme cases do you need to consider the most drastic and painful cure—a complete layoff. This is reserved for emergencies like being feverish or so sore that you can't run without limping.

The general rule for running after an injury or illness has occurred is this: If the symptoms decrease or disappear as you go, keep going. You probably aren't doing yourself further harm. But if the symptoms grow as you go, stop before you hurt yourself any more.

### • What exercises should I do besides running?

Dr. George Sheehan, the medical advisor for *Runner's World* magazine, says, "When you run, three things happen to your body. And two of them are bad."

The good one is that you become better at running. You build endurance and speed. But at the same time, your legs become overspecialized. Running is straight-ahead, every-step-the-same movement. So the muscles which lift the legs and drive them forward become strong. They also become tight.

These are the two bad things which happen when you run: The muscles in the back of the body—calves, hamstrings, buttocks and lower back—grow strong and inflexible. And the front muscles—shins, quadriceps and stomach—don't keep pace. A strength imbalance develops.

The tightness and imbalance increase as you become a better runner—and they increase the chances of injury. The most common of these injuries are knee pain, shin splints, achilles tendonitis, pulls of the calf or hamstring muscles and irritation of the sciatic nerve.

Corrective exercises can't solve all your injury problems, because injuries have a combination of causes (see previous question). But you can remove one of your aggravations by balancing running with strengthening and stretching.

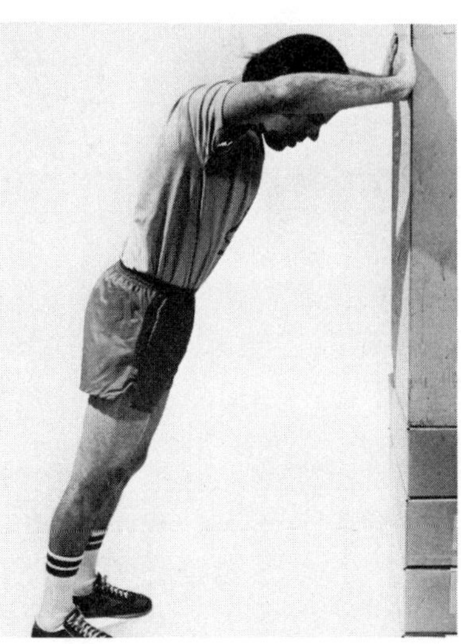

*Exercise One: wall pushup.*

First, test for trouble. Stand up straight, then try to bend over and touch the ground with your fingertips. That's the minimum standard for flexibility. Now lie down, make a bridge with your knees and try to do a bent-leg sit-up. Doing one without having anyone or anything hold your feet in place is the minimum standard of abdominal strength.

If you can pass the tests, keep exercising to maintain your adequate strength and flexibility. If you can't pass them, correct the deficiency before it gets worse.

Dr. Sheehan recommends six exercises, which he calls the "Magic Six." Three are stretches, three are strengtheners. They take about a minute each to do, and should be done at least once a day. Do them before or after running, or both.

The three flexibility exercises:

1. *Wall pushup* for calf muscles. Stand flat-footed about arms' length from a wall. Lean toward the wall until you start to hurt. Hold to count of 10, relax for 10 seconds, repeat the exercise two more times.

2. *Hamstring stretch.* Put your straightened leg up on a table, chair or other object which is about crotch high. Bend forward until you start to hurt. Hold to count of 10, relax 10 seconds, repeat the exercise two more times, then do the same with the other leg.

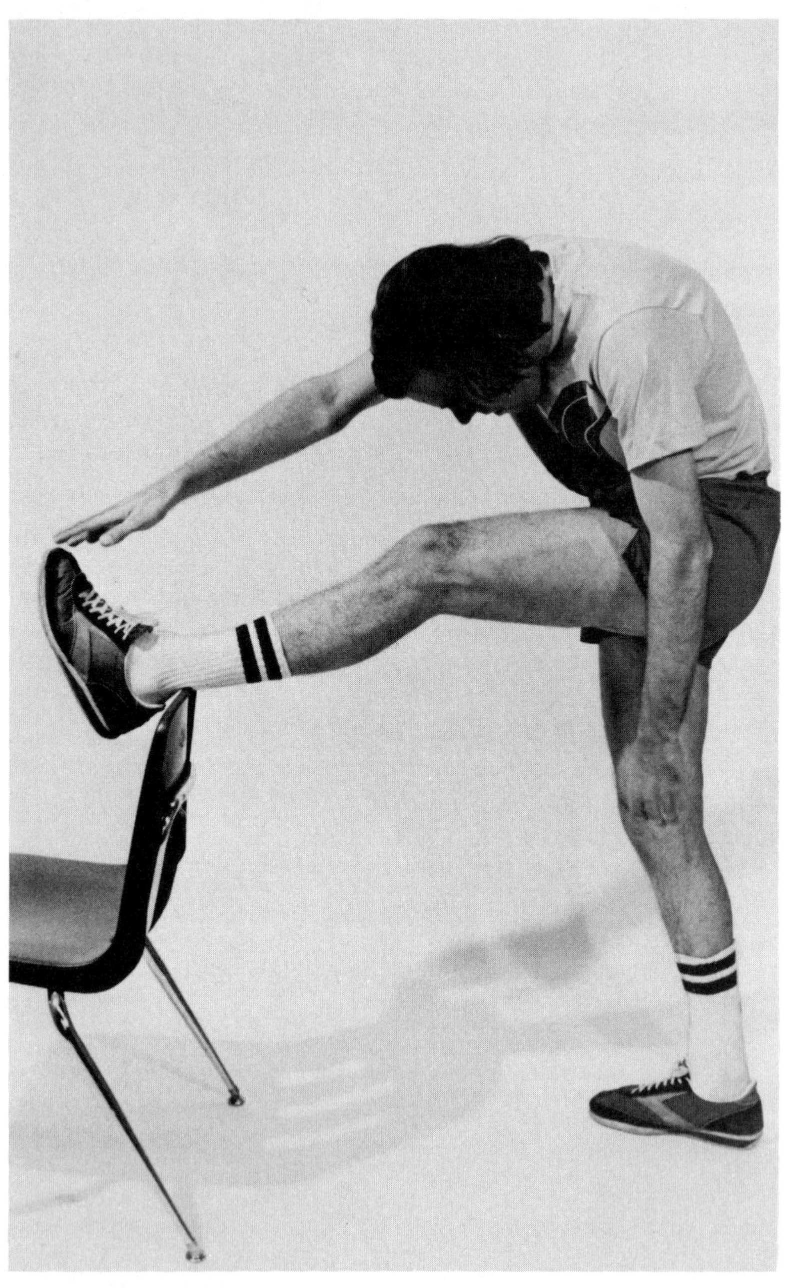

*Exercise Two: hamstring stretch.*

3. *Backover* for hamstrings and lower back. Lie on the floor, then bring straight legs over your head and down until you start to hurt. Hold to count of 10, relax 10 seconds, repeat the exercise two more times.

Now do the three strengthening exercises:

4. *Bent-leg sit-up* for abdominal muscles. Lie with knees bent and feet close to buttocks. Lift head and shoulders at least six inches off the ground. Repeat until you can't do any more sit-ups or have reached 20.

5. *Shin muscles.* Sit on a table or bench with legs hanging down. Put a light weight (five pounds or less) over the toes and flex the foot at the ankle. Hold to count of six, relax for six seconds, repeat the exercise four more times, then do the same with the other leg.

6. *Quadriceps (thigh) muscles.* Same position and weight as in exercise four. Straighten the leg, locking the knee. Hold to count of six, relax for six seconds, repeat the exercise four more times, then do the same with the other leg.

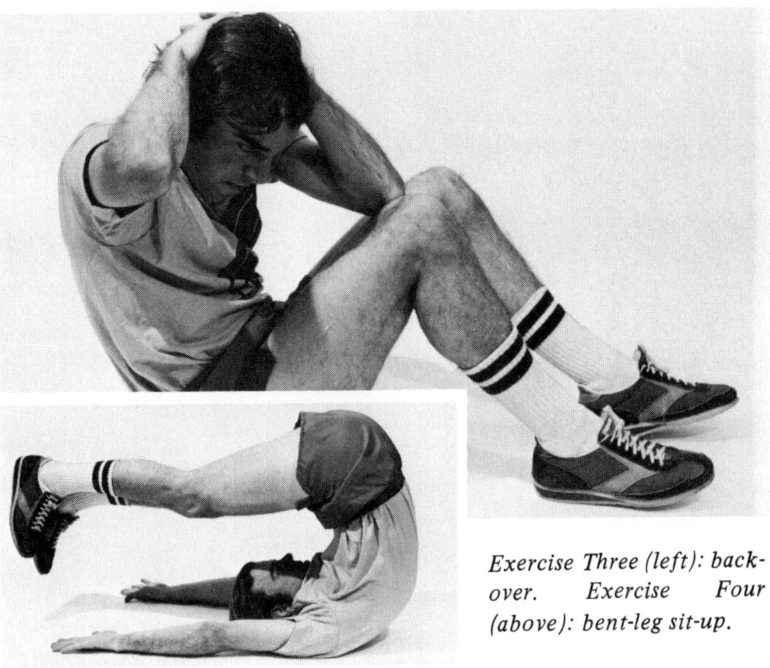

*Exercise Three (left): backover. Exercise Four (above): bent-leg sit-up.*

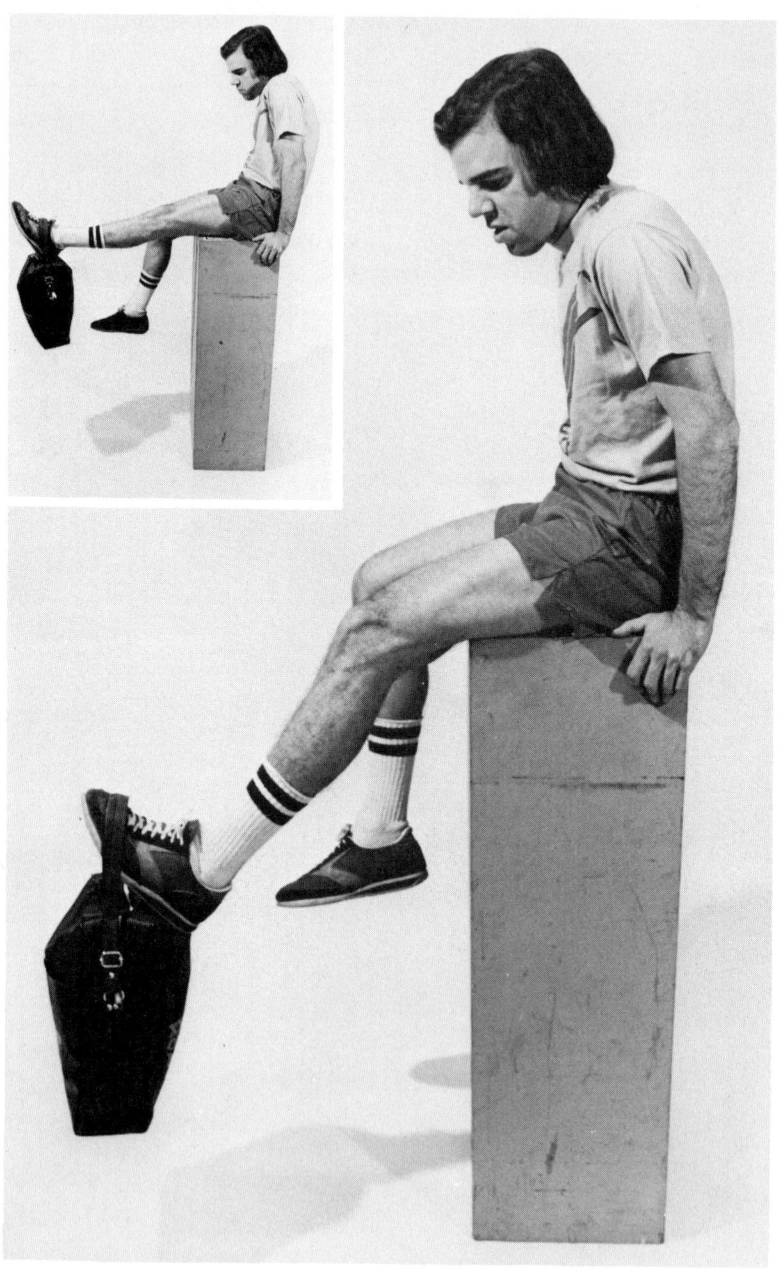

*Exercise Five (inset): shin muscles. Exercise Six: quadriceps muscles.*

# PART FIVE

# RACING

# Lesson 25

# Introducing Racing

Each new lesson throughout the book has represented a step up in experience and knowledge. Each new section has meant a shift in emphasis. I started with walking as remedial work leading up to jogging. Then came jogging for fitness, followed by running for fun. Now you are ready for training to race.

You may have raced before. But that wasn't more than a minor goal during the fun-running period. The race was a small, informal one, you did little specific preparation for it, and your expectations weren't very high. You simply were experimenting with racing.

Now you know. And if you're reading on into this section, there were things about racing which intrigued you. They sharpened your appetite for racing, and you're wanting to do more of it, more seriously.

This means you must start to train. I know I've used the word "train" before. It slips into my vocabulary where it doesn't belong sometimes, because I was raised on racing and learned to talk of all non-racing as "training." Actually, to train is to prepare for a future race. It is like the research writer does for his book or the rehearsal an actor does for his play. It is background work done solely as a means to an end.

By this definition, I don't "train" any more. Like most fun-runners, I run for today. Running is an end in itself, and if it gets me ready for a race tomorrow, that is just coincidence. I race, but I take a fun-runner's approach to it. I'm not serious

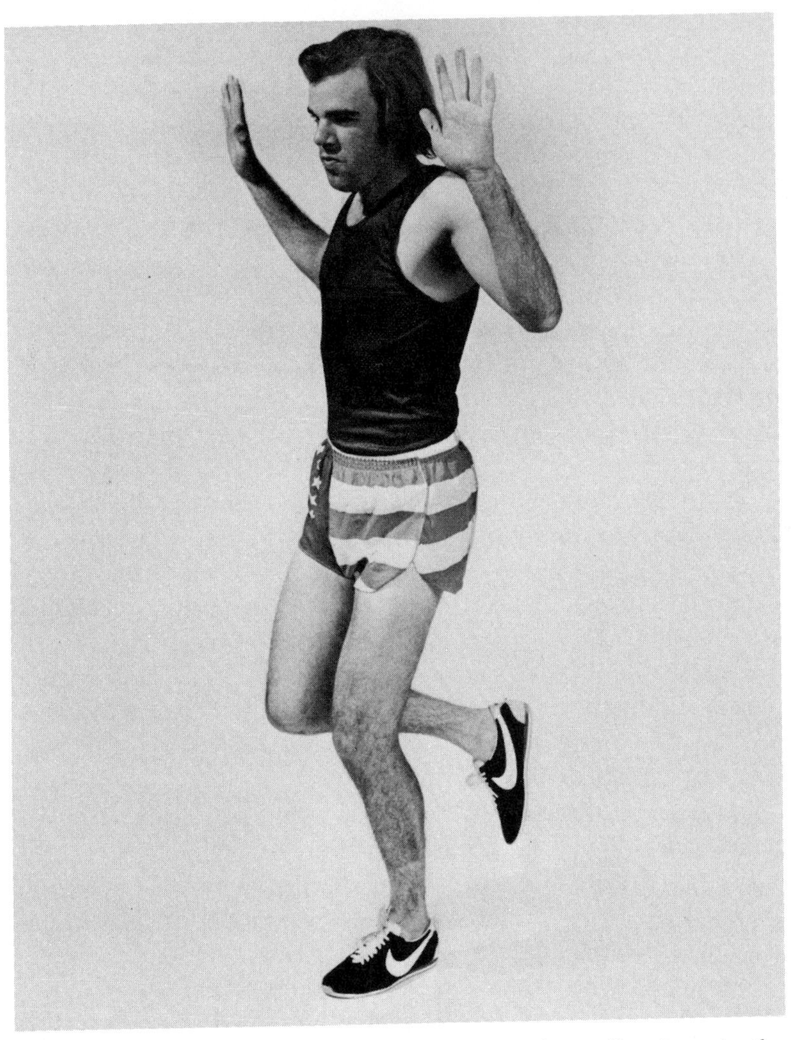

*"A newly-serious racer usually is drawn in one of two directions–to the marathon or the mile. These are the classic distances . . . ."*

enough to drive myself long distance at high speeds and risk spoiling the fun.

I'm not saying that fun and hard work are mutually exclusive. It's just a different type of satisfaction in racing–a more serious kind of fun which comes of making a commitment to excellence and carrying it through.

The excellence might come from long distances, high speeds

or a combination of the two. A newly-serious racer usually is drawn in one of two directions—to the marathon or the mile. These are the classic distances in running, and every runner knows their significance.

The first question asked of a marathoner is, "Did you finish?" and of a miler, "What time did you run?"

The marathon is the ultimate endurance test. Oh sure, people sometimes go longer than that. But 26 miles 385 yards is where racing ends and where ludicrous extremes begin.

The mile is the perfect test of prolonged speed. It is long enough to demand the intelligent pacing and tactics of a distance runner, but short enough that it requires the explosiveness of a sprinter.

You must train seriously for a marathon just to finish one, and in the finishing lies its satisfaction. Anyone who runs can finish a mile, but few of us can run one fast. Success in miling comes in improving your times—times whose meaning everyone knows.

Choose which you want to do—distance or speed. By training for a marathon, you'll be ready to race well at any distance above six miles. With mile training, you'll have the speed for any race a quarter-mile to six miles.

Now a split develops in training. The milers go one way, the marathoners the other. Milers go fast, marathoners long. But while the details of their training aren't the same, the general patterns are. It is, in fact, the same seasonal pattern which has trailed through the book from walking through racing: a break-in month, a build-up month and a speed-up month.

Before entering the new season, you will have satisfied several prerequisites:

1. You now have a score in the mid- to high 20s for the fitness test in Lesson Four.

2. You can run an "excellent" time for your age and sex in the 12-minute run described in Lesson 15.

3. You have raced with a group at least once, have finished the race and know you can handle more.

Once the new season starts, both miler and marathoner will follow a similar training week in that it mixes hard and easy, long and short days. But the days themselves will be quite different for the two types of runners.

• *Break-in.* Get used to doing more, whether the "more" is speed or distance.

If you're a miler, keep doing about as much distance as in the "running" season. But see that each day's run includes 5-10% speed. Add it, informally and untimed, after the longer, slower runs, and gradually work up to your expected mile pace. Run a short race or two to learn what that pace is.

If you're a marathoner, start increasing the distances, because you have a long way to go and not much time to get there. Work both on lengthening the longest run and lifting the daily average. Try a race in the 6-7-mile range to get the feel of going long and rather fast. Keep a few gentle accelerations in all the runs, throughout the season, for the sake of speed and leg looseness.

• *Build-up.* Your quickest increase in tempo or distance will come this month.

Milers, formalize your speedwork somewhat. Keep within the 5-10% ratio of speed to distance, but begin to time the fast running on a track, running at your current predicted mile pace. Race at least once, preferably at two or three miles.

Marathoners, get your mileage up to a minimum of 50 per week. Better yet, in the 60-70 range. And make the longest run of the week 15-20 miles. Race once at 10 miles or more.

• *Speed-up.* This is when you polish yourself for the big event. You've laid the foundation. Now finish the job.

Milers, cut down somewhat on your distance running. Do more racing or time-trialing, but save the important mile test until the end of the month. Run your speedwork at mile pace, but make your preliminary races a little shorter than a mile to feel the sensation of going a little faster.

Marathoners, level off in the mileage the first half of the month, then cut back as the race approaches. Early in the month, run a hard, fast race of 10-15 miles. Take the last long training run at least a week before the race. Be religious about taking a few short bursts of speed every day.

# Lesson 26

# Train Long

It's no secret that I am a pusher of LSD. My first book, written in 1969, was titled *LSD: The Humane Way to Train*, and I was using the stuff for several years before writing about it.

LSD in this case stands for "long, slow distance." And while I've been credited with developing it as a system of training and with coining the title, I claim credit for neither.

The name was lifted from the pages of *Long-Distance Log*. Browning Ross, a father of fun-running and road racing in the United States, needed to fill the bottom of a column one month. So he typed, "Use LSD—long, slow distance."

I liked it and applied it to what I already was doing. I was running rather long and slowly, and was putting in a lot of distance—as many people were beginning to do in the late 1960s.

I, like the others who were coming to the same conclusions independently, was slowing down and stretching out my runs for three main reasons: (1) as a reaction against excessive and painful speedwork; (2) to get ready to race at longer distances on the roads, since these events were growing in popularity then and (3) because running seemed more enjoyable when its pace was gentle.

I didn't originate this style of running. I just attached a name and a rationale to it in a slim, quickly produced little booklet. Its essential message was, "You don't have to hurt all the time or hate running to be good at it. You don't have to fight yourself. By running long and slowly, you stay healthy and happy, and you are able and eager to keep going. With regular running and an occasional race, you do pretty well."

There was some reaction against the message then, as there has been since. The criticism came from runners who didn't read the booklet very well, because their arguments aren't against what I've written.

Never, for instance, have I said LSD is the "best" way to train for maximum performance. As a training method, it is one good tool among many.

Never have I said that the LSD approach excludes all fast running. If you want to race, you have to do some running at race pace. My disagreement with hard-line trainers is only over the amount of "some" and when it should come. I think it doesn't need to total more than one mile in 10, and that most speedwork can be confined to the races themselves.

Never have I said that running LSD means plodding along all day at the slowest pace you can go while still satisfying the definition of "run." It's as inefficient to run too slowly as it is to go too fast. The best pace is one you can run comfortably.

Never have I set a specific time which is defined as "LSD pace." It's too variable and relative for that. Your own comfortable pace will improve as you get more fit, and it will change from day to day as you run through cycles of high energy and fatigue. It may even vary by a minute per mile or more within a single run. I know my own pace probably ranges from seven- to nine-minute miles each day.

Many of the leading runners make a point of saying, "I never do LSD-type running" when they talk of their training. And almost all of them do it, by my definition. That is, anything more than a minute per mile above race pace is LSD.

I can't race as fast as Frank Shorter or Bill Rodgers, the top two US marathoners, go in their training. But that doesn't mean our relative effort isn't the same. They race long distances at about five minutes per mile. If they train at six minutes, they're working no harder than I—a seven-minute racer—am when I run eight-minute miles. This theory of relativity doesn't take an Einstein to figure out.

I used to be bothered a little by criticisms of the way I ran, because they raised doubts in my own mind about whether it was right or not. I don't have those doubts any more. I know I'm doing what's right for me, and I am writing only for the people who choose to agree. I'll argue only to defend the integrity of our approach, not to win over any doubters.

My reasons for running this way are beyond argument by now. They are established facts which require no defense other than a simple listing of those facts:

1. *Gently-paced running is the safest and surest way to work up your distances.* If you're aiming for a marathon, you must do a certain amount of running to get ready for it. About 50 miles a week is a bare minimum. You're running about half that much now, so you're facing a doubling of time and effort. The only way you can absorb the extra load is to hold the pace down until you can cover the distance easily. Distance comes first, speed later.

My background was in speed. I was a high school and college miler, and when I was learning to run longer, that background turned against me. Despite my years of running, it was months before I could run 10 straight miles. I couldn't slow down enough to go long. I tried five marathons before I could finish one without walking. Same reason: running too fast to go long.

The first problem of a beginning marathoner–perhaps *any* marathoner–is learning to keep going, and speed gets in the way of that lesson.

2. *Speed can develop out of endurance.* There's a strange alchemy at work here, and you may have to suspend logic to understand it. I'm about to show how you can race faster by training slower, and this is the hardest LSD trick to believe.

It is based on the fact that speed is largely inherited and that not much can be done to improve it. We can polish our basic speed and can become more efficient at using it. But we waste our time by running always at top speed, thinking we will push the peak higher.

Better to work at it from the bottom. Work on endurance, because it can be improved to an incredible degree through training. We can't make ourselves go much faster at top speed, but we can extend the distances we run at high speeds by improving stamina. Stamina comes from longish, slowish running.

I was amazed when I started running long and slowly. My only ambition was to finish a marathon. The time was irrelevant, just so I made it. I trained solely for distance. I quit forever the kind of training I thought it took to be a track racer—interval 440s, time trials, five-mile "overdistance" workouts at red-line pace. The only time I ran faster than 7-8 minutes per mile was in races.

What amazed me was that most of the early-day suffering had been for nothing. My mile to six-mile times stayed as fast as before or were faster, just because I knew how to last.

3. *I keep doing it.* I started running this way without giving any thought to improving my racing times, and the surprising improvement has long since stopped. But I keep running every day in the same way I have since 1966, and lots of other runners have joined me since then. This is the best argument of all for the worth of LSD.

## Lesson 27

# Break In

### MILE TRAINING

Remember the rule: endurance first, speed later. You pick up much of your speed not by training fast but by increasing your staying power. You can't do much more than sharpen up the speed you were born with, but you can train yourself not to poop out so soon when you're going fast if you practice at distances a lot longer than a mile.

Distance runs at well below mile race pace will account for more than nine in 10 of your miles this month. Only in the last mile are you allowed to test your speed. This ratio summarizes the relative importance and placement of the two main elements of training.

As a fun-runner, you were up to running about 60 minutes or its mileage equivalent on your longest day each week, 40-45 minutes on the two medium-long days, and 20-30 minutes on the remaining short and easy days. Keep that up. There's no reason to increase it, but you don't want the amount of running to shrink, either. This is the endurance foundation on which speed is to be built. If you can't run 3-8 or more miles comfortably, you'll be limited in how fast you can cover a single one.

Start the month with a mile time trial by yourself. This will give you a starting point from which to improve your time, and it will tell you how mile race pace is supposed to feel.

Remember that pace and run a little of it every day from now on. You've accelerated during your long runs before, so you know how it's done (Lesson 28 has full details). Now make those bursts somewhat faster and do them after the long runs. Later in the month, start going to the track.

Finish the month with a "fun-run" type of mile race—with other people but without much seriousness attached to the setting or the result.

## MARATHON TRAINING

Twenty-six miles 385 yards still seems an incredible distance from your rather meager 3-8 mile runs. You have a long ways to go yet, it's true, but remember that you also have a long time to get there.

Just as I had three months to build this book up to 200 pages, you have three months to build yourself up to a marathon. I wrote a few pages at a time. You will add a few minutes at a time, starting immediately.

A tolerable increase in distance is about 10% a week. You're starting from a base of about a half-hour of running a day. Through 10% weekly jumps, you can have that up to 45 minutes by the month's end. You can push your longest run from 60 to 90 minutes. Maintain the same pattern of long (one day), medium (two days) and short (four days) as before, with long runs being 1½ times the average and short runs half of the average time or distance.

Do your brief accelerations during each day's run, but do them in a different way and for a different purpose than the miler does. Run only mildly fast, only to keep your legs from growing tight and rutted in a constant pace. These changes of pace should be energizing, not tiring.

End the month with a road race or time trial of at least a quarter-marathon (6.6 miles). Concentrate more on holding a faster-than-normal pace than on the final time and place.

## First Month's Mile Plan

| Day | Suggested Training | Actual Training |
|---|---|---|
| 1 | 20-minute run plus 2 x 30 seconds at race pace* | |
| 2 | 20-minute run plus 2 x 30 seconds at race pace | |
| 3 | 40-minute run plus 2 x one minute at race pace | |
| 4 | 20-minute run plus 2 x 30 seconds at race pace | |
| 5 | 40-minute run plus 2 x one minute at race pace | |
| 6 | 20-minute run plus 2 x 30 seconds at race pace | |
| 7 | Mile time trial** | |
| *Daily average for first week (31 minutes):* | | |
| 8 | 20-minute run plus 3 x 30 seconds at race pace | |

| Day | Suggested Training | Actual Training |
|---|---|---|
| 9 | 20-minute run plus 3 x 30 seconds at race pace | |
| 10 | 40-minute run plus 3 x one minute at race pace | |
| 11 | 20-minute run plus 3 x 30 seconds at race pace | |
| 12 | 40-minute run plus 3 x one minute at race pace | |
| 13 | 20-minute run plus 3 x 30 seconds at race pace | |
| 14 | One-hour run plus 3 x one minute at race pace | |
| *Daily average for second week (36 minutes):* | | |
| 15 | 20-minute run plus 3 x 220 yards*** | |
| 16 | 20-minute run plus 3 x 220 yards | |

| Day | Suggested Training | Actual Training |
|---|---|---|
| 17 | 40-minute run plus<br>3 x 440 yards | |
| 18 | 20-minute run plus<br>3 x 220 yards | |
| 19 | 40-minute run plus<br>3 x 440 yards | |
| 20 | 20-minute run plus<br>3 x 220 yards | |
| 21 | One-hour run plus<br>3 x 440 yards | |
| *Daily average for third week (36 minutes):* | | |
| 22 | 20-minute run plus<br>3 x 220 yards | |
| 23 | 20-minute run plus<br>3 x 220 yards | |
| 24 | 40-minute run plus<br>3 x 440 yards | |
| 25 | 20-minute run plus<br>3 x 220 yards | |
| 26 | 40-minute run plus<br>3 x 440 yards | |

| Day | Suggested Training | Actual Training |
|---|---|---|
| 27 | 20-minute run plus 3 x 220 yards | |
| 28 | mile race or time trial** | |
| *Daily average for fourth week (31 minutes):* | | |
| 29 | makeup day**** | |
| 30 | makeup day | |
| 31 | makeup day | |

*Total number of running days for month (28):* __________

*Total amount of running for month (950 minutes):* __________

*Average amount of running per day (34 minutes):* __________

(*run at approximately mile pace with relatively short recovery periods between; **warm up thoroughly for all races and time trials; ***run untimed on the track or another measured course; 220 yards is a half-lap of a standard track, 440 yards is a full lap; ****make up for sessions missed during the month)

# First Month's Marathon Plan

| Day | Suggested Training | Actual Training |
|---|---|---|
| 1 | 25-minute run* | |
| 2 | 25-minute run | |
| 3 | 45-minute run | |
| 4 | 25-minute run | |
| 5 | 45-minute run | |
| 6 | 25-minute run | |
| 7 | Quarter-marathon race or time trial** | |
| *Daily average for first week (34 minutes):* | | |
| 8 | 25-minute run | |
| 9 | 25-minute run | |
| 10 | 50-minute run | |
| 11 | 25-minute run | |
| 12 | 50-minute run | |
| 13 | 25-minute run | |
| 14 | 1:10 run | |
| *Daily average for second week (38 minutes):* | | |

| Day | Suggested Training | Actual Training |
|---|---|---|
| 15 | 30-minute run | |
| 16 | 30-minute run | |
| 17 | 50-minute run | |
| 18 | 30-minute run | |
| 19 | 50-minute run | |
| 20 | 30-minute run | |
| 21 | 1:20 run | |
| *Daily average for third week (43 minutes):* | | |
| 22 | 30-minute run | |
| 23 | 30-minute run | |
| 24 | 1:00 run | |
| 25 | 30-minute run | |
| 26 | 1:00 run | |
| 27 | 30-minute run | |
| 28 | 1:30 run | |
| *Daily average for fourth week (47 minutes):* | | |

| Day | Suggested Training | Actual Training |
|---|---|---|
| 29 | makeup day*** | |
| 30 | makeup day | |
| 31 | makeup day | |
| *Total number of running days for month (28)* | | |
| *Total amount of running for month (1135 minutes):* | | |
| *Average amount of running per day (40 minutes):* | | |

(*it is recommended that about 5% of each day's run be done at faster than normal pace; this amounts to three minutes per hour; **a quarter-marathon is slightly more than 6½ miles; ***make up for sessions missed during the month)

# Lesson 28

# Train Fast

"Long, slow runs have a lot of things going for them, but I don't think injury prevention is one of them."

The man in the audience wasn't saying this for the sake of argument. I'd run with him several mornings that week, and we seemed to agree on the way we like to run.

Now I was in front of the crowd, answering questions about the gentle style of running. He had stood to ask a question. He wasn't challenging me. He simply wanted an answer to a problem of his.

He said, "I love to run LSD. But I seem to get hurt *more* often, not less. For instance, every time I try to race, I'm at least very sore for several days afterward. And often I hurt my achilles tendons, calves or knees. The sudden changes from very slow to very fast running seems to be too much of a shock on the legs. Do you think at least a little bit of speedwork is necessary to get used to the stresses of racing?"

I said, "Yes, you have a good point there. It may be possible to race *too seldom* as well as too often. Racing too often can exhaust you and break you down. But if you race too seldom, you may not be up to handling the 'shock,' as you put it.

"This is why I say that about 5% of the total miles should be at racing pace. It seems to be about the ideal ratio, at least for me. It's enough to keep me ready to race without tearing my legs apart, but not so much that it grinds me down.

"So, to answer your question in a round-about way, if you're racing regularly—about one mile in every 20—I don't think you

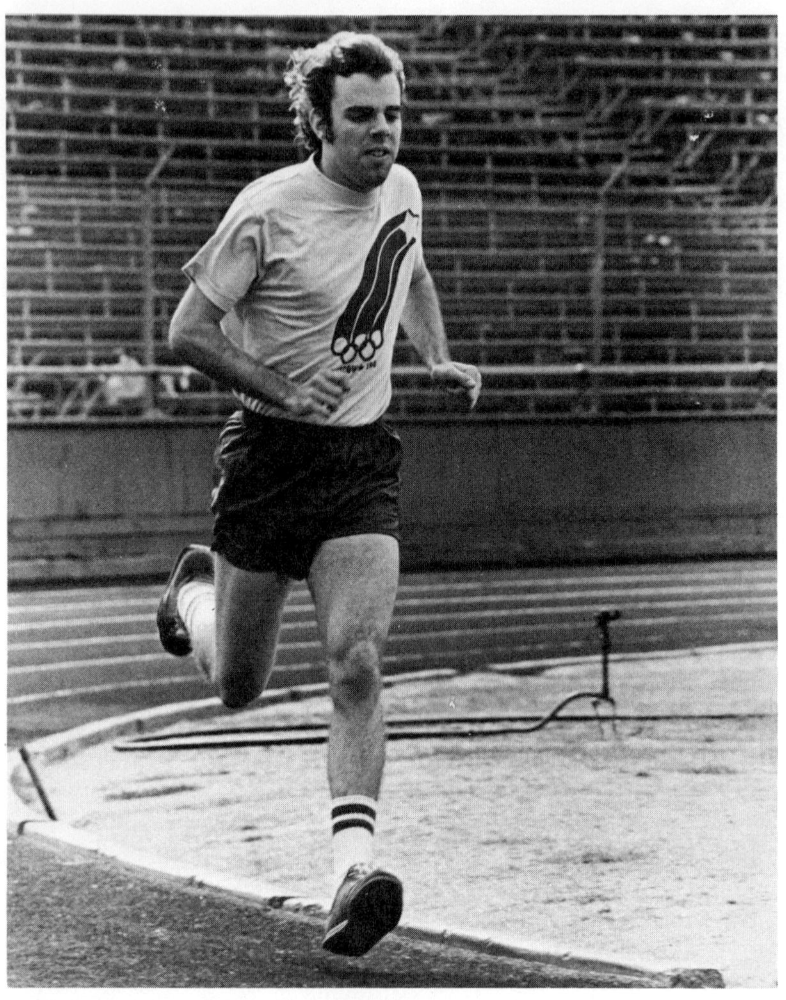

*"Accelerate and decelerate gently, reach out and drive powerfully but smoothly, get the feeling of relaxed speed . . . ."*

need any supplementary speedwork in training. But if you've gone long periods between races, you may want to do one of two things to be safe: (1) run a couple of 'break-in' races at less than full speed to get yourself used to this kind of stress again, or (2) add a few short, non-exhausting speed runs to your training."

I was talking down to him, talking as if I had all the answers and he had none, and talking in the abstract. As I look back on the exchange now, I see that this runner and I had gone through the same things, and he had learned faster than I had. I had raced and been hurt because I hadn't followed either of the recommended paths. There had never been a "break-in" race. Every race was all-out. And I'd never done anything but slow running on all the other days since August 1966.

In recent months I'd seen something else which seemed to go against my cherished theories about running. I hurt when I *didn't* race. When I went a long time without running fast, my calves, achilles tendons, heels and knees took on a dull, stiff soreness. Racing sometimes corrected it.

It's clear to me now that it wasn't the race itself which loosened me up. More often, one set of pains was replaced by another after racing. The reason the race was therapeutic was that it got me up off my heels and stretched out muscles which had been moving only through a narrow, stereotyped range. A gentler kind of fast running does the same things without the same risks that racing has.

Running authority Hal Higdon has written, "Perhaps the most cogent comment I can make on speed training is that the top runners use it too much and the bottom runners use it too little . . . . My advice would be that the speed runners do less and the slow runners do more, and maybe we'll all meet in the middle."

And when we arrive, maybe we'll find Dr. Ernst van Aaken already is there. Dr. van Aaken is the German physician-coach-researcher-theoritician whose book, *The Van Aaken Method*, I edited. It was a hell of a job. The doctor is a far better thinker and doer than writer, for one thing. He writes in paragraph-long sentences which are as confusing as his method is simple. He repeats and sometimes even contradicts himself.

There were days when I was so disgusted with the whole mess that I could have sent it out the back door to the garbage bin. But in the end I was happy with the book and happier that I'd worked so closely with it. Easy jobs are never examined. They're done quickly, then forgotten. *Van Aaken* wasn't easy, so I had to study it word by word.

Van Aaken taught me how to run fast without self-destructing. He set the ideal ratio of endurance to speed running at about 20:1–20 easy miles for every hard one. It doesn't mean taking the speed miles in one racing bash followed by a long recovery period, as I once thought. Van Aaken's is a "pay-as-you-go" plan.

Previously I had taken my weekly or monthly 5% all at once, gone deeply into debt and then spent the rest of the week or month bailing myself out. It was as if I were doing stretching exercises only a few times a month. I'd forget how to stretch from one session to the next. And I'd make each session so long and violent that I'd need a long time to get over the soreness.

I know I can't do this with stretching. I must stretch a little bit every day to stay loose. I should have known that the same is true of speed. Fitness doesn't come from once-in-a-while torrents of hard work, but from regular dribbles of moderate effort.

Van Aaken has known this for decades. That's why his runners go through a full range of movements each day–mostly gentle running, but with some walking and faster dashes, too. His Germans end their long runs with mini speed sessions. These are no more than one-twentieth (5%) of the total distance, no faster than the pace of one's race, no more than one-fourth the racing distance and are never exhausting.

Dr. van Aaken is a scientist. He is precise in the running he prescribes. The speed sessions are formalized, on the track, measured and timed. I'm more haphazard about my running. So while I agree completely with the doctor on the proper combination of endurance and speed, I combine them in a somewhat different way.

I'm way past the point of doing anything in running just because it's good for me. I don't run 100-mile weeks or go 20-plus miles on Saturdays or train twice a day or carbo-load or guzzle athletic drinks to gain a few seconds of time. And I won't add speed just for that reason. Racing fitness alone isn't enough to justify it. It must be a plus in terms of the overall pleasure I get from running. There are enough minuses conspiring to stop me without adding a new one.

The first test of anything new I add to my running is, "Did I start doing it without first asking is it worth doing?"

The speed supplement passed this test. One day in February, near the end of an hour's run, I simply started. I didn't plot it out in advance. I didn't think what it might mean to the immediate health of my legs or to my future racing.

It was spontaneous and instinctive. A voice in me shouted "go!" and I went. I accelerated for a minute or so, slowed down to jog for a while, sped up again, slowed, sped. That was enough. The voice which had urged me on was quiet now. I felt loose and exhilarated.

I'm an hour-a-day runner. One-twentieth (5%) of an hour is three minutes. So I now add three minutes of faster running to my usual long and slow runs. It's blended right in without a break, and is done wherever I happen to be at the moment.

The idea here is to accelerate and decelerate gently, to reach out and drive powerfully but smoothly, to get the feeling of relaxed speed.

This speed plan has evolved:

1. Continue to run the same distances as always. These are based, in my case, on the longest distance I plan to race.

2. Insert the fast runs at will, after a thorough warmup of slow running. I like to do mine in the last half of my sessions.

3. Do the pickups at about the pace of the fastest race.

4. Fall back into normal, gentle pace after each pickup. Recover fully before starting the next one.

5. Run fast for only 5% of the total training time–one minute in every 20. I find it is easiest to use a "three of something" approach. In a 30-minute run, I insert three 30-second pickups; in an hour run, three one-minutes; in two hours, three two-minutes. This works out to a precise 5%.

6. Don't do the pickups when muscles and tendons are painful and faster running increases the pain. More likely the speeding will have the opposite effect. It has for me.

My muscles and tendons seldom are sore now, which is reason enough to speed a little. I didn't start it to race faster but I'm doing that, too. I run a half-mile fun-run every few weeks as a speed test. The times have improved by an average of 10 seconds since Dr. van Aaken got his point across.

# Lesson 29

# Build Up

## MILE TRAINING

Become more specific in your running this month. Keep doing about the same amount of distance running (an average of about 40 minutes a day) and the same percentage of speed (5-10% of the total), but now do it closer to the place and the pace of the race. Run speed training on the track, if possible, and time the fast bursts.

The speed still will only amount to one minute for every 20 minutes of slower running. But now you make it a more formal minute. End the distance run at the track (or a similar flat, measured course only if no track is available). Walk a few minutes before starting the timed laps, and walk until recovered if you're taking more than one burst.

Run 440 (one lap) or 220 yards (half-lap) at your current best mile pace. For instance, if you did 5:20 in your last mile time trial or race, run the laps in 80 seconds. Run three 440s on the "long" and "medium" days, and three 220s on the "short" days.

Don't race any miles this month, because you want to stay hungry now for this distance. Instead, build some specific racing stamina by running in events of two and three miles. These teach you to hold a fast pace for two or three times your target distance, and will make it seem shorter and easier later.

## MARATHON TRAINING

The goals for the month are these: (1) run more than two

hours straight; (2) race 10 miles, and (3) push up your "collapse-point" training level. The first two are pretty straightforward, but the last takes more explaining.

"Collapse-point" is the theoretical distance at which a runner has to slow down drastically or stop. His training won't take him any farther. This point is somewhere near three times the average distance he runs each day.

Obviously, then, a marathoner-to-be wants to work his training mileage up to the point where he is averaging at least a third of a marathon each day. That way, a "collapse" isn't likely to occur.

A third of a marathon is slightly less than nine miles—or 60-70 minutes of running time. You will be averaging that amount by the middle of the month.

Keep following the schedule which moves you ahead by a steady, sensible 10% per week. During the month, the short runs progress to 40-45 minutes, the medium ones to 80-90 minutes and the long ones past two hours.

Continue to add modest bursts of speed during all runs to give the legs some variety and stretch. Insert three of these fast spurts, each about as long in seconds as the total run is in minutes (for example, 80 seconds during an 80-minute session). This gives you a perfect 5% speed supplement.

Race 10 miles or more at the pace you hope someday to carry through a full marathon.

## Second Month's Mile Plan

| Day | Suggested Training | Actual Training |
|---|---|---|
| 1 | 20-minute run plus 3 x 220 yards* | |
| 2 | 20-minute run plus 3 x 220 yards | |
| 3 | 40-minute run plus 3 x 440 yards | |
| 4 | 20-minute run plus 3 x 220 yards | |
| 5 | 40-minute run plus 3 x 440 yards | |
| 6 | 20-minute run plus 3 x 220 yards | |
| 7 | One-hour run plus 3 x 440 yards | |
| *Daily average for first week (36 minutes):* | | |
| 8 | 20-minute run plus 3 x 220 yards | |
| 9 | 20-minute run plus 3 x 220 yards | |
| 10 | 40-minute run plus 3 x 440 yards | |
| 11 | 20-minute run plus 3 x 220 yards | |

| Day | Suggested Training | Actual Training |
|---|---|---|
| 12 | 40-minute run plus 3 x 440 yards | |
| 13 | 20-minute run plus 3 x 220 yards | |
| 14 | 3-mile race or time trial ** | |
| *Daily average for second week (31 minutes):* | | |
| 15 | 20-minute run plus 3 x 220 yards | |
| 16 | 20-minute run plus 3 x 220 yards | |
| 17 | 40-minute run plus 3 x 440 yards | |
| 18 | 20-minute run plus 3 x 220 yards | |
| 19 | 40-minute run plus 3 x 440 yards | |
| 20 | 20-minute run plus 3 x 220 yards | |
| 21 | One-hour run plus 3 x 440 yards | |
| *Daily average for third week (36 minutes):* | | |

| Day | Suggested Training | Actual Training |
|---|---|---|
| 22 | 20-minute run plus 3 x 220 yards | |
| 23 | 20-minute run plus 3 x 220 yards | |
| 24 | 40-minute run plus 3 x 440 yards | |
| 25 | 20-minute run plus 3 x 220 yards | |
| 26 | 40-minute run plus 3 x 440 yards | |
| 27 | 20-minute run plus 3 x 220 yards | |
| 28 | two-mile race or time trial** | |
| *Daily average for fourth week (31 minutes):* | | |

| Day | Suggested Training | Actual Training |
|---|---|---|
| 29 | makeup day*** | |
| 30 | makeup day | |
| 31 | makeup day | |

*Total amount of running days for month (28):*__________

*Total amount of running for month (950 minutes):*__________

*Average amount of running per day (34 minutes):*__________

(*run the 220s and 440s on the track and time them, attempting to run a bit faster each week but no faster than current mile racing ability; **warm up thoroughly for all races and time trials; ***make up for sessions missed during the month)

## Second Month's Marathon Plan

| Day | Suggested Training | Actual Training |
|---|---|---|
| 1 | 35-minute run* | |
| 2 | 35-minute run | |
| 3 | 1:10 run | |
| 4 | 35-minute run | |
| 5 | 1:10 run | |
| 6 | 35-minute run | |
| 7 | 10-mile race or time trial | |
| *Daily average for first week (50 minutes):* | | |
| 8 | 35-minute run | |
| 9 | 35-minute run | |
| 10 | 1:10 run | |
| 11 | 35-minute run | |
| 12 | 1:10 run | |
| 13 | 35-minute run | |
| 14 | 1:50 run | |
| *Daily average for second week (56 minutes):* | | |

| Day | Suggested Training | Actual Training |
|---|---|---|
| 15 | 40-minute run | |
| 16 | 40-minute run | |
| 17 | 1:20 run | |
| 18 | 40-minute run | |
| 19 | 1:20 run | |
| 20 | 40-minute run | |
| 21 | 2:00 run | |
| *Daily average for third week (63 minutes):* | | |
| 22 | 45-minute run | |
| 23 | 45-minute run | |
| 24 | 1:30 run | |
| 25 | 45-minute run | |
| 26 | 1:30 run | |
| 27 | 45-minute run | |
| 28 | 2:00 run or more | |
| *Daily average for fourth week (69 minutes):* | | |

| Day | Suggested Training | Actual Training |
|---|---|---|
| 29 | makeup day** | |
| 30 | makeup day | |
| 31 | makeup day | |

*Total number of running days for month (28):*____________

*Total amount of running for month (1660 minutes):*________

*Average amount of running per day (59 minutes):*__________

(*it is recommended that about 5% of each day's run be done at faster than normal pace; this amounts to three minutes per hour; **make up for sessions missed during the month)

# Lesson 30

# Put It Together

This is a lesson on race pacing, and it's one I've learned twice. I've had two lives as a runner—first as a trackman and later as a road racer. And very early in each of those lives, I learned that I was not indestructible.

I wrote somewhere earlier about my first race as a miler. I was 14 years old, a freshman in high school, and was out to show the bigger and older boys how this race is run. No matter that I'd been running less than a week and had never gone a full mile before. Something told me I was a born miler, the way other boys are born to be football and basketball stars.

The start was like a panicked rush to escape a burning movie house. I had to sprint out with everyone else to keep from being crushed. Even going as fast as I could, I dropped nearly to last place on the backstretch. I tried to tell myself, "Don't worry. They're going too fast, and they'll come back to me."

But I wasn't kidding myself. I was the one who was falling back, going too fast and worrying. After a little more than a lap—the fastest lap I'd ever run—I dropped out.

Years later, I ran my first long-distance race on the roads. I'd satisfied most of my ambitions as a miler and was looking for something new to do. The marathon was it.

At the time, I still was making the transition from speed to distance. I was averaging no more than four or five miles a day. But when a chance came to run 30 kilometers, I took it. Thirty kilometers is a little less than 19 miles, and it also was then about three times as far as I'd ever raced.

"No problem," I said as I entered. "As long as I go slow enough, I can make it."

The trouble was, I didn't start slowly. It felt slow enough because I was used to the mad dash of the mile. We seemed to be plodding the early miles of the long race, and I grew impatient. I stretched out and began to pass people. The more I passed, the more I stretched.

By 10 miles, I was in the top 10 places. The pace was below six minutes per mile, and I was wondering, "What's so hard about this kind of running?"

A mile later, I found out. We rounded a corner and ran into a hill. It was so tall and steep that it looked like a sheer face. I meant to keep running, but my legs rebelled. I didn't feel the kind of pain I'd known from the mile. My head was clear, but its messages weren't getting past my waist. I eventually finished, but only by combining walking with a pathetic shuffling imitation of a run. I didn't walk normally again for a week.

These two first races taught me the same two lessons:

- One is that the most important part of a race is run before the race begins. That is in the training for it. In the case of the mile, I had done no training worthy of that description. Before the first road race, I hadn't done nearly enough. My background had, at best, prepared me to go about 12 miles—and the first race was half-again longer than that.
- The second lesson was to start cautiously, saving something for the real racing which begins after the halfway point. In my first mile and first marathon-like race, I was run out before the racing began.

You have the advantage of knowing in advance the things I had to run badly to learn. So you'll be able to avoid most or all of my first-race pain and frustration.

Whether you're a miler or a marathoner, you will have done the needed preparation before the race. The schedules here will have led you through enough distance training and then a small but adequate amount of speedwork.

You will have built the race into yourself. Then all you'll have left to do is bring it out. You'll bring distance and speed together and to the surface with the right kind of pacing.

A crusty old coach once told me, "You've paced yourself right if you used your last drop of energy in the last step of the race. Any race you can walk away from was not a good one."

I'm not asking you to judge your racing that severely, because if I did I'd have to judge my own that way. And it would mean I've only run four or five good races in more than 500. But the old coach did make one important point. He said pacing was a matter of spreading available reserves over the distance to be raced, neither running dry too soon nor having too much left at the end.

Novice racers seldom have trouble spending everything they have. Their problem is the opposite one—pooping out early. This happens because they almost always err in the direction of too much speed, too soon, instead of too slow of a start.

If someone starts this way because he doesn't know any better (as I did), I can excuse him. But I'm not leaving you with any excuse. I want to drum the word, the meaning and the practice of pace into you so completely that you'll never ruin a race by starting it like an Olympian and finishing it (if you finish) like a first-day jogger. Races are too precious to waste that way.

There are three steps in pace learning—one to study, one to practice in training and one to use in the race itself.

1. *Study.* Learn the meaning of "splits." Those are the intermediate times given during races, usually at each lap of the mile and every five miles during the marathon. The most efficient way to use energy during a race is to make your split times as even as possible.

The accompanying charts show what even-pace times are for the mile and marathon. Memorize them so you'll know what they mean when they're shouted at you. Allow for a little variation to account for normal pacing patterns. In the mile, the first and fourth laps usually are a little faster than the middle ones. Marathoners run fairly steadily through 20 miles then slow a bit from there to the end.

2. *Practice.* Develop a "feel" for pace by timing yourself occasionally during training, and by running low-key races at your

favorite and other distances. Experienced runners come to have a clock in their head which tells them within seconds how fast they are going. This is valuable in races where you aren't carrying a stopwatch and where checkpoints may be as much as five miles apart.

3. *Apply.* Divide the race into two parts, holding back during the first and whipping yourself on during the second.

A well-known coach from New Zealand, Arthur Lydiard, once wrote, "The best way to get the full benefit of ability in the mile is to go out with the attitude that it is a half-mile race and, as far as you are concerned, the time to start putting on pressure is when the first half-mile is behind you."

Lydiard wasn't recommending a *slow* start so much as a *controlled* one. He realizes what every runner must: that you can't win a race early, but you can blow it there. This is true of every race. To hold a steady pace means ever-increasing effort. At first it seems too easy, but as you go along you must run harder and harder just to stay where you are.

Kenny Moore, two-time US Olympic marathoner, tells how this works in his event: "To be effective over the last six miles, one must harbor some sort of emotional as well as physical reserve. An intense, highly competitive frame of mind over the early part of the run seems to evaporate at 20 miles. So I prefer to begin in a low-key sort of yawning-sleepy state of semi-consciousness. I watch the scenery and the other runners with appreciation rather than with any sort of competitive response. I chat with anyone so inclined.

"Later, entering the last six miles, I get enthusiastic about racing. A strong acceleration gives me a lift, and I can usually hold a new rhythm to the finish. It's more fun to pass people late in the race where it means something. The last six miles is the stage where I try honestly to use everything I have left. That, of necessity, hurts."

# 1-6-Mile Pacing

| 440 | Mile | 2 Miles | 3 Miles | 4 Miles | 5 Miles | 6 Miles |
|---|---|---|---|---|---|---|
| 57 | 3:48 | | | | | |
| 58 | 3:52 | | | | | |
| 59 | 3:56 | | | | | |
| 1:00 | 4:00 | | | | | |
| 1:01 | 4:04 | | | | | |
| 1:02 | 4:08 | 8:16 | | | | |
| 1:03 | 4:12 | 8:24 | | | | |
| 1:04 | 4:16 | 8:32 | 12:48 | 17:04 | | |
| 1:05 | 4:20 | 8:40 | 13:00 | 17:20 | | |
| 1:06 | 4:24 | 8:48 | 13:12 | 17:36 | 22:00 | 26:24 |
| 1:07 | 4:28 | 8:56 | 13:24 | 17:52 | 22:20 | 26:48 |
| 1:08 | 4:32 | 9:04 | 13:36 | 18:08 | 22:40 | 27:12 |
| 1:09 | 4:36 | 9:12 | 13:48 | 18:24 | 23:00 | 27:36 |
| 1:10 | 4:40 | 9:20 | 14:00 | 18:40 | 23:20 | 28:00 |
| 1:11 | 4:44 | 9:28 | 14:12 | 18:56 | 23:40 | 28:24 |
| 1:12 | 4:48 | 9:36 | 14:24 | 19:12 | 24:00 | 28:48 |
| 1:13 | 4:52 | 9:44 | 14:36 | 19:28 | 24:20 | 29:12 |
| 1:14 | 4:56 | 9:52 | 14:48 | 19:44 | 24:40 | 29:36 |
| 1:15 | 5:00 | 10:00 | 15:00 | 20:00 | 25:00 | 30:00 |
| 1:16 | 5:04 | 10:08 | 15:12 | 20:16 | 25:20 | 30:24 |
| 1:17 | 5:08 | 10:16 | 15:24 | 20:32 | 25:40 | 30:48 |
| 1:18 | 5:12 | 10:24 | 15:36 | 20:48 | 26:00 | 31:12 |
| 1:19 | 5:16 | 10:32 | 15:48 | 21:04 | 26:20 | 31:36 |
| 1:20 | 5:20 | 10:40 | 16:00 | 21:20 | 26:40 | 32:00 |
| 1:21 | 5:24 | 10:48 | 16:12 | 21:36 | 27:00 | 32:24 |
| 1:22 | 5:28 | 10:56 | 16:24 | 21:52 | 27:20 | 32:48 |
| 1:23 | 5:32 | 11:04 | 16:36 | 22:08 | 27:40 | 33:12 |
| 1:24 | 5:36 | 11:12 | 16:48 | 22:24 | 28:00 | 33:36 |
| 1:25 | 5:40 | 11:20 | 17:00 | 22:40 | 28:20 | 34:00 |
| 1:26 | 5:44 | 11:28 | 17:24 | 22:56 | 28:40 | 34:24 |
| 1:27 | 5:48 | 11:36 | 17:36 | 23:12 | 29:00 | 34:48 |
| 1:28 | 5:52 | 11:44 | 17:48 | 23:28 | 29:20 | 35:12 |
| 1:29 | 5:56 | 11:52 | 17:48 | 23:44 | 29:40 | 35:36 |
| 1:30 | 6:00 | 12:00 | 18:00 | 24:00 | 30:00 | 36:00 |
| 1:31 | 6:04 | 12:08 | 18:12 | 24:16 | 30:20 | 36:24 |
| 1:32 | 6:08 | 12:16 | 18:24 | 24:32 | 30:40 | 36:48 |
| 1:33 | 6:12 | 12:24 | 18:36 | 24:48 | 31:00 | 37:12 |
| 1:34 | 6:16 | 12:32 | 18:48 | 25:04 | 31:20 | 37:36 |
| 1:35 | 6:20 | 12:40 | 19:00 | 25:20 | 31:40 | 38:00 |
| 1:36 | 6:24 | 12:48 | 19:12 | 25:36 | 32:00 | 38:24 |
| 1:37 | 6:28 | 12:56 | 19:36 | 25:52 | 32:20 | 38:48 |
| 1:38 | 6:32 | 13:04 | 19:36 | 26:08 | 32:40 | 39:12 |
| 1:39 | 6:36 | 13:12 | 19:48 | 26:24 | 33:00 | 39:36 |

# 5-50-Mile Pacing

| Mile | 5 Miles | 10 Miles | 15 Miles | 20 Miles | Marathon | 50 Miles |
|---|---|---|---|---|---|---|
| 4:50 | 24:10 | 48:20 | 1:12:30 | 1:36:40 | 2:07:44 | |
| 5:00 | 25:00 | 50:00 | 1:15:00 | 1:40:00 | 2:11:06 | |
| 5:10 | 25:50 | 51:40 | 1:17:30 | 1:43:20 | 2:15:28 | |
| 5:20 | 26:40 | 53:20 | 1:20:00 | 1:46:50 | 2:19:50 | |
| 5:30 | 27:30 | 55:00 | 1:22:30 | 1:50:00 | 2:24:12 | |
| 5:40 | 28:20 | 56:40 | 1:25:00 | 1:53:20 | 2:28:34 | |
| 5:50 | 29:10 | 58:20 | 1:27:30 | 1:56:40 | 2:32:56 | |
| 6:00 | 30:00 | 1:00:00 | 1:30:00 | 2:00:00 | 2:37:19 | 5:00:00 |
| 6:10 | 30:50 | 1:01:40 | 1:32:30 | 2:03:20 | 2:41:41 | 5:08:20 |
| 6:20 | 31:40 | 1:03:20 | 1:35:00 | 2:06:40 | 2:46:03 | 5:16:40 |
| 6:30 | 32:30 | 1:05:00 | 1:37:30 | 2:10:00 | 2:50:25 | 5:25:00 |
| 6:40 | 33:20 | 1:06:40 | 1:40:00 | 2:13:20 | 2:54:47 | 5:33:20 |
| 6:50 | 34:10 | 1:08:20 | 1:42:30 | 2:16:40 | 2:59:09 | 5:41:40 |
| 7:00 | 35:00 | 1:10:00 | 1:45:00 | 2:20:00 | 3:03:33 | 5:50:00 |
| 7:10 | 35:00 | 1:11:40 | 1:18:20 | 2:23:20 | 3:07:55 | 5:58:20 |
| 7:20 | 36:40 | 1:13:20 | 1:50:00 | 2:26:40 | 3:12:17 | 6:06:40 |
| 7:30 | 37:30 | 1:15:00 | 1:52:30 | 2:30:00 | 3:16:39 | 6:15:00 |
| 7:40 | 38:20 | 1:16:40 | 1:55:00 | 2:33:20 | 3:21:01 | 6:23:20 |
| 7:50 | 39:10 | 1:18:20 | 1:57:30 | 2:36:40 | 3:25:23 | 6:31:40 |
| 8:00 | 40:00 | 1:20:00 | 2:00:00 | 2:40:00 | 3:29:45 | 6:40:00 |
| 8:10 | 40:50 | 1:21:40 | 2:02:30 | 2:43:20 | 3:34:07 | 6:48:20 |
| 8:20 | 41:40 | 1:23:20 | 2:05:00 | 2:46:40 | 3:38:29 | 6:56:40 |
| 8:30 | 42:30 | 1:25:00 | 2:07:30 | 2:50:00 | 3:42:51 | 7:05:00 |
| 8:40 | 43:20 | 1:26:40 | 2:10:00 | 2:53:20 | 3:47:13 | 7:13:20 |
| 8:50 | 44:10 | 1:28:20 | 2:12:30 | 2:56:40 | 3:51:35 | 7:21:40 |
| 9:00 | 45:00 | 1:30:00 | 2:15:00 | 3:00:00 | 3:56:00 | 7:30:00 |
| 9:10 | 45:50 | 1:31:40 | 2:17:30 | 3:03:20 | 4:00:22 | 7:38:20 |
| 9:20 | 46:40 | 1:33:20 | 2:20:00 | 3:06:40 | 4:04:44 | 7:46:40 |
| 9:30 | 47:30 | 1:35:00 | 2:22:30 | 3:10:00 | 4:09:06 | 7:55:00 |
| 9:40 | 48:20 | 1:36:40 | 2:25:00 | 3:13:20 | 4:13:28 | 8:03:20 |
| 9:50 | 49:10 | 1:38:20 | 2:27:30 | 3:16:40 | 4:17:50 | 8:11:40 |

# Lesson 31

# Speed Up

## MILE TRAINING

You're closing in on the mile now. The racing becomes more frequent and faster, much of the training simulates racing, and your distance running is little more than a warmup for the speedwork to follow.

Race twice in low-key half-miles, so you'll know the feeling of moving faster than you will in a mile. This will make mile pace seem less of a strain to maintain. Put less emphasis on overall times in these "halves" than on going steady and fast.

Twice a week, run simulated mile races. Go the full mile for time, but run only two of the laps at all-out mile pace, the other two about 15 seconds slower. One day, push the first and third laps while coasting the second and fourth. Another day, switch the order–first and third fast, second and fourth easier.

For instance, if you plan to run a five-minute mile, equal laps are 75 seconds each. In the simulated run, two laps are 75 but the others are 90. This works out to a mile of 5:30, or about 90% of top speed.

Take these runs on your medium-hard days, following a gentle half-hour lope. On the weekly long-run day, go about an hour and finish with three paced 440s, same as last month. On short days, run about 20 minutes, then do two brisk 220s, the second faster than the first.

Taper down in the last week before the big race by running just 20-30 minutes easily and 2-3 fast half-laps each day.

## MARATHON TRAINING

You've gone as far as you should go without doing an extra month or two of buildup. The distances in the schedule are all you need for now. They have peaked and will hold steady for the first two weeks of this month before shrinking away as race day approaches.

Run a half-marathon race or time trial early in the month. Then at mid-month, begin the long taper leading to the marathon. No training done in the last two weeks will make you more fit for the race, but overdoing it now can hurt. Cut back and gather strength for the big effort.

Don't bother to point out an obvious discrepancy in the program to me. I'm aware of it and can explain it. The marathon is 26-plus miles and requires 3-4 hours of running time, yet the schedule hasn't called for anything longer than two hours or about 15 miles. How are you supposed to make up the difference?

Trust me. You'll make it up in the race because you have run enough total distance. It is the total amount of running which determines how far you can go, not the length of your longest runs. If you've averaged 60-70 minutes a day in training, you can go three times that long. You'll see.

Running too far in practice causes two problems. First, it can be exhausting. It can wipe out the next week's training, costing you hours of work for a few extra minutes of running. Second, it can be depressing. You may go 20 or more painful miles by yourself and think, "The race is going to be even worse."

Leave the hardest part of the marathon unexplored until race day. Then let the other runners help carry you through it.

## Third Month's Mile Plan

| Day | Suggested Training | Actual Training |
|---|---|---|
| 1 | 20-minute run plus 2 x 220 yards* | |
| 2 | 20-minute run plus 2 x 220 yards | |
| 3 | 30-minute run plus "simulated mile" (first and fourth laps at racing pace, others 15 seconds slower each) | |
| 4 | 20-minute run plus 2 x 220 yards | |
| 5 | 30-minute run plus "simulated mile" (same pattern as Day 3) | |
| 6 | 20-minute run plus 2 x 220 yards | |
| 7 | Half-mile race or time trial** | |
| *Daily average for first week (29 minutes):* | | |
| 8 | 20-minute run plus 2 x 220 yards | |
| 9 | 20-minute run plus 2 x 220 yards | |

| Day | Suggested Training | Actual Training |
|---|---|---|
| 10 | 30-minute run plus "simulated mile" (laps one and three at race pace, others 15 seconds slower each) | |
| 11 | 20-minute run plus 2 x 220 yards | |
| 12 | 30-minute run plus "simulated mile" (same pattern as Day 10) | |
| 13 | 20-minute run plus 2 x 220 yards | |
| 14 | One-hour run plus 2 x 440 yards | |
| *Daily average for second week (34 minutes):* | | |
| 15 | 20-minute run plus 2 x 220 yards | |
| 16 | 20-minute run plus 2 x 220 yards | |
| 17 | 30-minute run plus "simulated mile" (laps two and four at race pace, others 15 seconds slower each) | |
| 18 | 20-minute run plus 2 x 220 yards | |

| Day | Suggested Training | Actual Training |
|---|---|---|
| 19 | 40-minute run plus "simulated mile" (same pattern as Day 17) | |
| 20 | 20-minute run plus 2 x 220 yards | |
| 21 | Half-mile race or time trial** | |
| *Daily average for third week (29 minutes):* | | |
| 22 | 20-minute run plus 2 x 220 yards | |
| 23 | 20-minute run plus 2 x 220 yards | |
| 24 | 20-minute run plus 2 x 220 yards | |
| 25 | 20-minute run plus 2 x 220 yards | |
| 26 | 20-minute run plus 2 x 220 yards | |
| 27 | 20-minute run plus 2 x 220 yards | |
| 28 | mile race** | |
| *Daily average for fourth week (26 minutes):* | | |

| 29 | makeup day*** | |
|---|---|---|
| 30 | makeup day | |
| 31 | makeup day | |

*Total number of running days for month (28):*__________

*Total amount of running for month (815 minutes):*__________

*Average amount of running per day (29 minutes):*__________

(*220s and 440s are run on the track or other measured courses, and are timed; **warm up thoroughly before all races and time trials; ***make up for sessions missed during the month)

# Third Month's Marathon Plan

| Day | Suggested Training | Actual Training |
|---|---|---|
| 1 | 45-minute run* | |
| 2 | 45-minute run | |
| 3 | 1:30 run | |
| 4 | 45-minute run | |
| 5 | 1:30 run | |
| 6 | 45-minute run | |
| 7 | Half-marathon race or time trial** | |
| *Daily average for first week (64 minutes):* | | |
| 8 | 45-minute run | |
| 9 | 45-minute run | |
| 10 | 1:30 run | |
| 11 | 45-minute run | |
| 12 | 1:30 run | |
| 13 | 45-minute run | |
| 14 | 2:00 run or more | |
| *Daily average for first week (69 minutes):* | | |

| Day | Suggested Training | Actual Training |
|---|---|---|
| 15 | 30-minute run | |
| 16 | 30-minute run | |
| 17 | 1:00 run | |
| 18 | 30-minute run | |
| 19 | 1:00 run | |
| 20 | 30-minute run | |
| 21 | 1:30 run | |
| *Daily average for third week (47 minutes):* | | |
| 22 | 30-minute run | |
| 23 | 30-minute run | |
| 24 | 30-minute run | |
| 25 | 30-minute run | |
| 26 | 30-minute run | |
| 27 | 30-minute run | |
| 28 | Marathon race | |
| *Daily average for fourth week (55 minutes):* | | |

| Day | Suggested Training | Actual Training |
|---|---|---|
| 29 | makeup day*** | |
| 30 | makeup day | |
| 31 | makeup day | |

*Total number of running days for month (28):*__________

*Total amount of running for month (1650 minutes):*__________

*Average amount of running per day (59 minutes):*__________

(*it is recommended that about 5% of each day's run be done at faster than normal pace; this amounts to three minutes per hour; **a half-marathon is 13.1 miles; ***make up for sessions missed during the month)

# Lesson 32

# Questions

- **What do I do right before the race?**

I'm not sure I have all the answers about what you should do, but I know some of the don'ts:

1. Don't eat yourself out of the race.

2. Don't be too worried about being worried.

3. Don't spend too little effort warming up if you're a miler or too much if you're a marathoner.

Pre-race diet is like pre-race training. Nothing you do in the last few hours is going to do you any good for the race, but it isn't too late to do yourself harm.

If you're normal, you're nervous before a race. Some people compulsively reach for food when they're nervous. Others feel weak and tired from tension and honestly think they need the energy which food can give. Everyone has trouble digesting food when worried. So the last few hours before a race is a particularly risky time to be eating.

Avoid it if you can. If you don't feel at all hungry, just don't eat. As Coach Arthur Lydiard has said, he's seen thousands of races and he's never seen anyone collapse from malnutrition yet. You aren't going to faint if you haven't eaten anything since the night before. But you might cramp up or throw up if you force something down.

If you are hungry, put something light and bland into the empty spot. A couple of pieces of toast or a few crackers, washed down by water or weak tea might do.

When I say it's normal to get nervous, this doesn't make it any less painful. It only helps you understand what is going on. Racing is hard work, harder work than you can do under normal circumstances. Your body has to call up its reserves to handle it. Nervousness is working to get you ready. It is clearing the wastes from your bladder and bowels, and taking attention away from the gut, out to the extremities. It is making your heart best faster and making you more alert, so you can react quickly and forcefully to the coming emergency.

You're on an emotional roller coaster. One minute, you can't wait for the race to begin. The next minute, you wish it would never come and you wish you could be anywhere else but here. Your physical feelings run parallel to these. First, you are ready to explode with energy. Then you wonder whether you have the strength to carry yourself to the bathroom one more time. You won't enjoy these things. But don't try to fight them, either. They're working for you.

Nervousness begins to fade as warmup begins. In the case of the miler, his warmup is longer than the race itself and is an essential preliminary round. Without it, he penalizes himself many seconds.

The race is so short and so fast that you don't get loose during its running. A complete warmup takes as much as a half-hour, and this race lasts only about five minutes. So you need what amounts to a workout before the mile. Run 20-30 minutes easily, then change into racing shoes and do two 220s at full racing pace. It's better to enter the race a little tired than a little cold and stiff.

If you're a marathoner, however, you may want to start your race a little cold and stiff. Take no warmup at all, and simply use the first half-hour of your race for loosening up. I say this because the biggest threat to a first marathon is starting too fast, and a cold start removes some of that temptation.

- **What kinds of problems can I expect to have during the race?**

The troubles with the mile come from its intensity–so much action packed into so little time. The marathon is complicated because there is so much distance and time in which things can go wrong.

First, the mile. One obvious fact of the race is that it is run on an oval track with two turns per lap. If there are lots of other people in the race with you, and you habitually run to the outside of them on the turns, you aren't running a mile any more. You may be going 30 yards farther. This is up to five seconds of running time—lost time.

On the other hand, you can lose time by hugging the curb and letting other runners to the front and outside box you in. Your first duty is to stay out of traffic congestion, even if it means going a few extra yards. You must maintain an empty running corridor ahead of you.

Once you have the room, stay to the inside all you can. Do most of your passing on the straightaways. If you have to go around someone on a turn to hold your momentum, swing out and back in quickly. Protect your precious seconds.

An all-out mile run taxes your breathing so heavily that you go deeply into "oxygen debt." This causes most of the physical stress you have to deal with during the race. By the second lap, your throat and chest are burning as you try vainly to suck up enough air to feed your hard-working muscles. The growing shortage of oxygen sets off chemical changes which begin to clog the muscles with fatigue products. By the third lap, your legs and arms have grown heavy, stiff and uncoordinated from the buildup of lactic acid. By the last lap, you're fighting off paralysis.

Running in oxygen debt hurts, and there's no way to avoid the hurting. What you do in preparing yourself for the race and pacing yourself through it is learn to manage the debt and not to panic when you go into the red.

The problems of running a marathon are altogether different than those in the mile. One track is pretty much like any other, but every road course is different. Hills, for example, make a course tougher and slower than the same distance would be if it were flat. If possible, choose a first-marathon course with little climbing. You have enough to worry about without adding this handicap.

Weather, too, is a major concern. In a mile, wind, cold or rain can kill a good time. Marathoners, however, need cool weather and are happy for breezes and rain which help in the cooling. Their enemy is heat, and "hot" for a marathoner can be anything above 60 degrees.

You can't control the weather, but you can plan a first race during a time of year when heat is unlikely. If the day is even mildly warm, plan to drink on the run. Take small amounts of liquid (a cup of water, special athletic drink or both), and take it frequently (every 20-30 minutes). Practice drinking during long training runs to be sure you can handle it.

Unlike in the mile, almost no oxygen debt develops in marathon running. There isn't the same sudden, sharp, sometimes severe pain that track runners feel. Rather, it is an overall numbness which comes on gradually with the miles of pounding.

Other runners don't get in your way as they do in the mile, because there is room on the open road for everyone. In the early miles, while you're fresh, you talk with them. Later, as you grow numb, you draw the strength to go on from the knowledge that they look as bad as you feel.

- **How do I recover after a race?**

By stages, and there are more of those stages than you may realize.

The first is acute discomfort. As soon as you stop, whether the race has been a mile or a marathon, you are nearly overwhelmed by the pains you've tried to ignore for the last several minutes or miles. Milers bend over, hands on their knees, hanging their heads and gasping to repay their oxygen debts. Marathoners who had run 26-plus miles now have a hard time persuading their legs to carry them to the nearest spot to sit down.

A miler should walk as soon as he is able, then after he changes shoes he should jog for a while to help pump the lactic acid from his muscles. A marathoner won't be able to do much, if any, post-race jogging. But he should at least do some walking around and stretching to keep from tightening up too quickly. In both cases, they shouldn't wait too long before putting on warmer clothes, because an overworked body chills and stiffens rapidly. Take a hot bath soon after racing, and enjoy a hot, self-indulgent meal after that.

For a day or two after a mile and several days after a marathon, you'll feel like you have a hangover. This is partly fatigue,

## The Spacing of Racing

Average Running Time Per Day

| Race Distance | 20 min. | 30 min. | 40 min. | 50 min. | 60 min. | 70 min. |
|---|---|---|---|---|---|---|
| mile | 3 days | 2 days | 2 days | 2 days | 2 days | 2 days |
| 2 miles | 5 days | 4 days | 3 days | 2 days | 2 days | 2 days |
| 3 miles | 9 days | 7 days | 5 days | 4 days | 3 days | 3 days |
| 6 miles | 20 days | 14 days | 10 days | 8 days | 7 days | 6 days |
| 10 miles | | 20 days | 15 days | 12 days | 10 days | 9 days |
| Half-Mar. | | | 23 days | 18 days | 15 days | 15 days |
| 15 miles | | | 27 days | 21 days | 18 days | 15 days |
| 20 miles | not recommended | | | 30 days | 25 days | 21 days |
| Mar. | | | | | 34 days | 29 days |

*Minimum recovery time recommended from one race to the next—based on 10 times distance of race; allow at least days for all.*

partly muscle soreness, partly psychological letdown which is inevitable after working so hard. Don't attempt to do any serious training during this time. Allow more recovery time than you think is necessary, because full recovery takes a lot longer than most people think.

Recovery from soreness is only the second of four stages. Muscle aches normally peak the second day after the race, then are gone after three or four days, and they may not even occur after a short race.

The third stage might be called "chemical recovery." This involves building back your energy reserves. They are moderately drained by the mile and severely depleted by the marathon, resulting in a listless, "blah" feeling. You may need as little as a few days or as much as a few weeks to return to normal.

The final stage of recovery is psychological. Experienced runners say, "You aren't ready to think about another race until you've forgotten how bad the last one felt." This may take weeks for a miler, months for a marathoner.

A good rule of thumb for insuring all levels of recovery is this: allow at least 10 easy minutes of recovery running for every minute of the race.

# Lesson 33

# Moving On

I'm a lifer. I've run on many more of my days than not, and I see nothing that will stop me from running on most of the days I have remaining.

Running makes up no more than one-twenty-fourth of each of these days. It is not something I crave constantly when I'm not doing it, the way a junkie barely exists from one fix to the next. It simply is a habit, a pleasant habit like eating a satisfying meal or sleeping through the night. I don't think much about it when it comes along right on schedule each day, but I miss it when it's no longer there.

I run for the same reasons I eat and sleep. Because I feel better when I do it than when I don't. Because regular exercise, like regular food and rest, is a physical and psychic need. It doesn't store well and the supplies are quickly used up, so they must be replaced nearly every day.

Running does no good if it doesn't last. After a few months away from it, even a world record holder or Olympic champion is no more of a runner than the next slob on the street.

Jim Ryun, the world's best miler in the 1960s, once took a long time off. He bulged to nearly 200 pounds (up 40 from his racing weight), and when he returned to training he couldn't run a five-minute mile. However, within a year he was running at record pace again.

Vladimir Kuts never again tried to become the runner he once had been. The Soviet was the scourge of the tracks in the 1950s, winning two gold medals in the '56 Olympics.

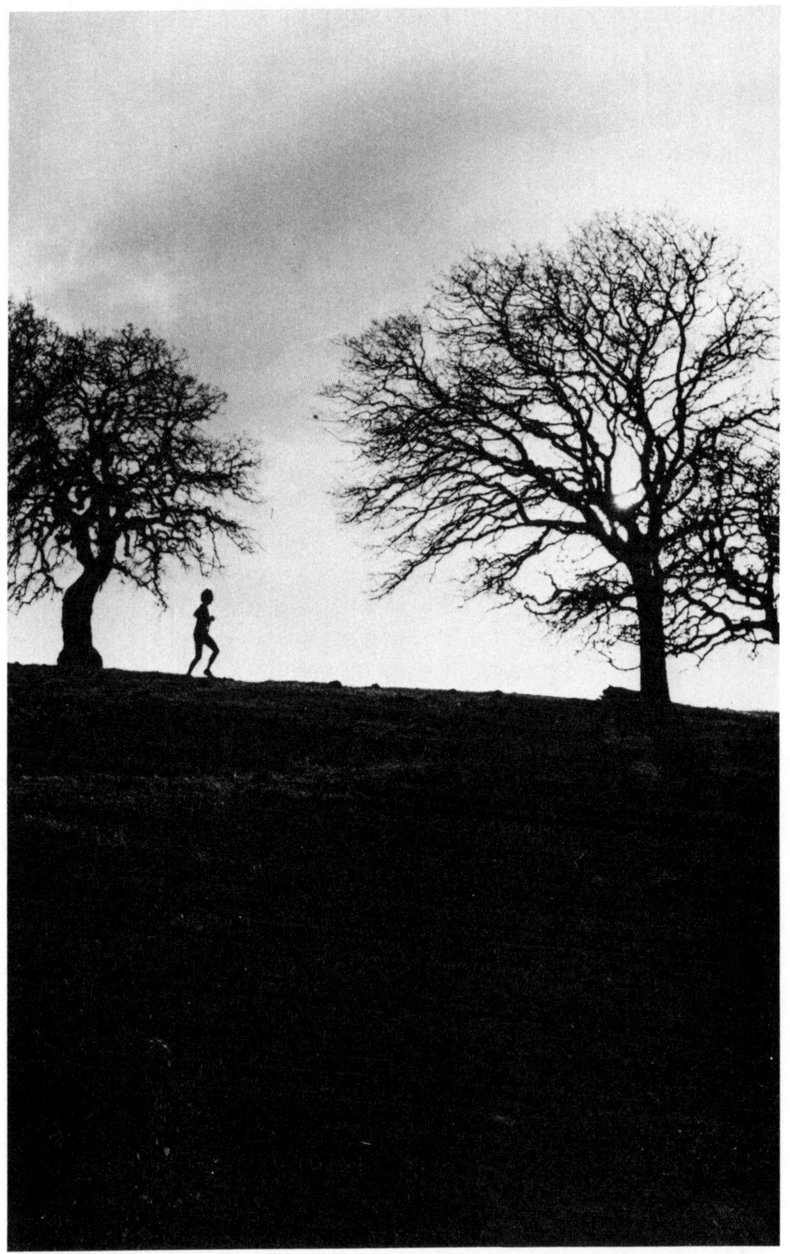

*"Too much physical stress, too much psychological tension, too many goals unmet are the reasons why runners become ex-runners . . . ."*

Other gold medalists have replaced Kuts, and his records are long since gone. When he quit racing, he quit running, too. He gained nearly 100 pounds. Kuts died at the age of 48.

I'm not saying that running is the road to immortality. Vladimir Kuts might have died of a heart attack at 48 even if he had kept running the extra 20 years. The sad thing in his, as in lots of less-publicized cases, was that he seemed so anxious to get rid of an activity which apparently had been good to him. Something in the way he approached his running wouldn't let him go on once his racing success was past.

Because I like to run and want to keep liking it enough to do it, I've quit holding star racers like Kuts in awe. Instead, I look at them to see what toll their success is taking and have promised myself I won't imitate them in ways which might limit my longevity as a runner.

Too much physical stress, too much psychological tension, too many goals unmet are the reasons why runners become ex-runners. This is why I take a rather conservative approach to training and racing. I don't ever want to stop.

I'm a lifer, and my only aim in writing is to make a lifer out of you. I wrote this book only to point you in certain directions, to help you develop a habit of everyday exercise, to teach some of the basics, to expose you to some of the opportunities and joys in running. You should know enough now to go on without me. Where you explore and evolve from here is up to your motivation and imagination.

# Recommended Reading

The following books and booklets all supply further information and advice on the topics covered in *Jog, Run, Race.* These publications, plus a listing of hundreds more, are available from World Publications, Box 366, Mountain View, Calif. 94042. Write for a current catalog.

*The Complete Runner*
*Dr. Sheehan on Running,* by George Sheehan, M.D.
*Encyclopedia of Athletic Medicine,* by George Sheehan, M.D.
*Exercises for Runners*
*The Long-Run Solution,* by Joe Henderson
*Racing Techniques*
*The Runner's Diet*
*Runner's Training Guide*
*Running with the Elements*
*Running with Style*
*The Van Aaken Method,* by Ernst van Aaken, M.D.
*Women's Running,* by Joan Ullyot, M.D.

World Publications also issues *Runner's World,* a monthly magazine which covers the sport in vivid detail. And the company promotes Fun-Runs. These informal events are conducted every Sunday morning of the year at the original site, Foothill College in Los Altos Hills, Calif., and at dozens of other places in the United States and abroad. A full list of sites is published each month in *Runner's World* and is available to anyone on request.

# About the Author

Joe Henderson exaggerates only slightly when he says, "I can't remember ever being a beginner." He began at age 14, nearly 20 years ago, in his native Iowa. And he hasn't stopped for more than a few days at a time since then.

Henderson's running and writing careers have paralleled each other. He raced in track and cross-country through high school and college, and at the same time was contributing news articles on the sports to local newspapers.

As a staff writer with *Track and Field News* and then editor of *Runner's World*, Henderson has been able both to watch running explode in participation and to report on the explosion. He perhaps is the most prolific running writer ever, having published hundreds of articles in addition to his nine books and booklets.

Henderson, who lives in Los Altos, Calif., with his wife Janet and daughter Sarah, continues to run his gently-paced hour a day because "I've long since forgotten how to stop."

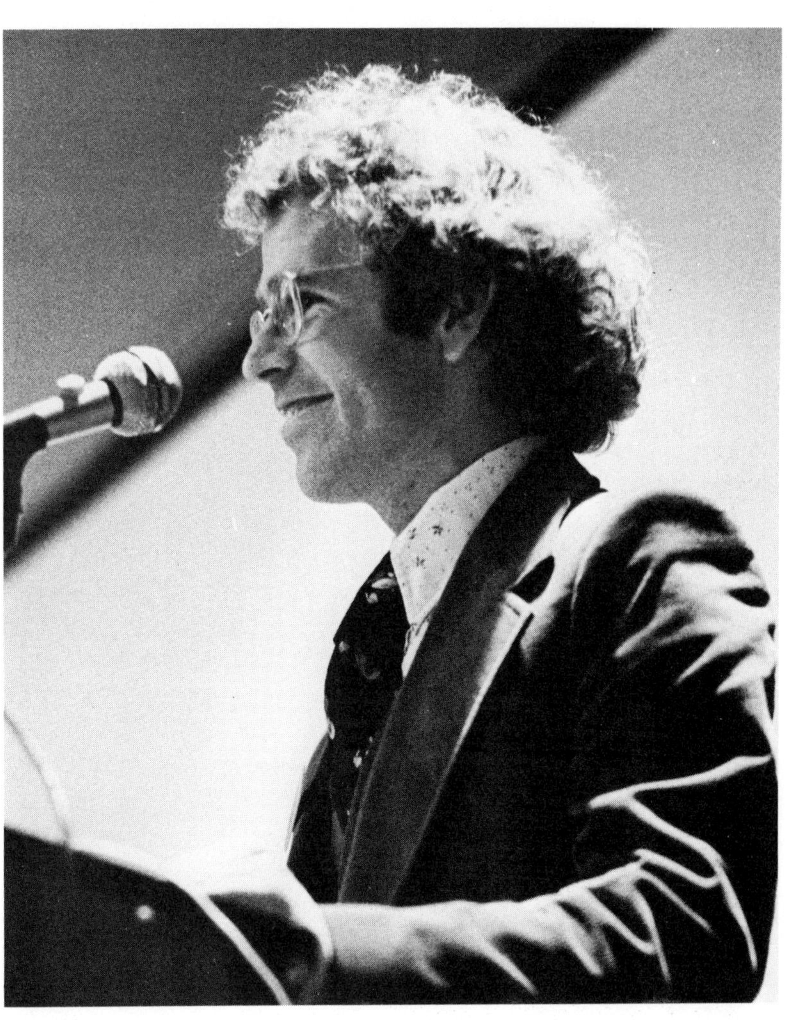